ABOUT THE AUTHORS

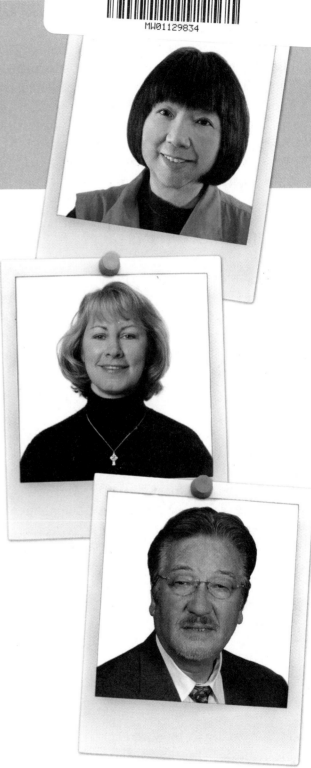

Audrey Yasukawa, MOT, OTR/L, CKTI

Audrey Yasukawa, OT, Certified Kinesio® Taping Instructor, is currently Chief of Occupational Therapy at LaRabida Children's Hospital. She previously served as a Resource Clinician at The Rehabilitation Institute of Chicago and assisted in the Upper Extremity Botox Clinic. Audrey piloted several pediatric research projects while at RIC and has published numerous articles on casting and taping. She has worked with adult and pediatric patients with a variety of neurological and orthopedic diagnoses. She is pediatric and adult NDT trained. She has over twenty years experience with upper extremity casting. Audrey has taught pediatric and adult taping courses internationally.

Patricia Martin, PT, CKTI

Patricia Martin, PT (Trish), Certified Kinesio® Taping Instructor, is currently Manager of Satellite Therapy Services at The Cleveland Clinic Children's Hospital, Shaker Campus. She previously worked in private practice and at Metro Health Medical Center treating adult and pediatric patients with a variety of diagnoses. These included TBI, SCI, CVA, and orthopedic issues. Trish has over twenty years of experience. She assists Beverly Cusick in courses on lower extremity biomechanics, splinting and casting and is pediatric NDT trained. She has taught pediatric and adult taping courses internationally.

Kenzo Kase, DC

Founder of the Kinesio® Taping Method
President of Kinesio® Taping Association
President of National Chiropractic College in Japan,
Director of the Japan Chiropractic Society
Vice President of Japan Sepaktakraw Federation under Japan Olympic Committee

Education:
- 1964- Meiji University, Tokyo, Japan- Bachelor of Arts in Business Administration.
- 1974- National College of Chiropractic, Chicago, Illinois- Doctorate of Chiropractic Medicine.
- 1978- Tokyo Acupuncture and Moxibustion Judo Therapist College- Certified Acupuncture and Moxicustion Therapist.

Dr. Kenzo Kase invented and developed the Kinesio® Taping Method nearly 30 years ago. The Kinesio® Taping Method is designed to facilitate the body's natural healing process while allowing support and stability to muscles and joints without restricting the body's range of motion. It successfully treats a variety of orthopedic, neuromuscular, neurological and medical conditions.

The method originated in Japan in 1973 and over the years it has stretched its horizons to countries worldwide. Today the method is used in countries such as: North, Central and South America, Australia, India, Africa and most of the European and Asian countries. Nearly 1,200 instructors are teaching this method to practitioners through out the world. Currently, the method is being used by occupational and physical therapists, athletic trainers, chiropractors, acupuncturists, and other health care practitioners alike.

Dr. Kase still teaches his method and continues to be active in the evolution of the technique and product.

TABLE OF CONTENTS

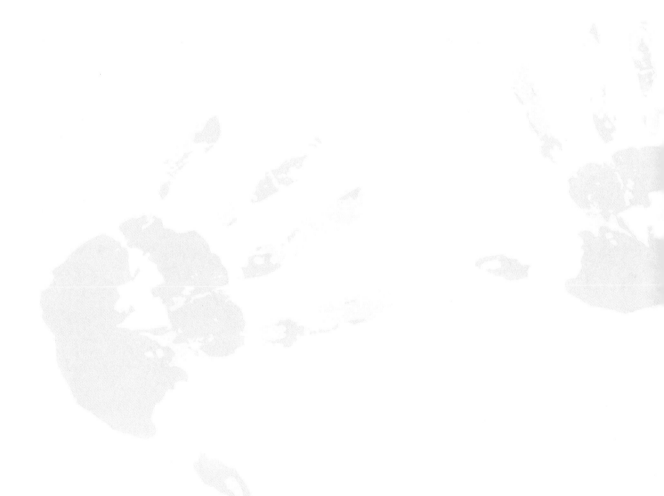

221 Diagnosis Specific Taping

241 Appendix

PREFACE

We have had the opportunity to study under the guidance of many talented instructors; Heather Murray, Ruth Coopee, Jim Wallis, and Ken Lamm. The Kinesio® Taping techniques introduced to us were primarily adult focused for pain management, sports, and rehabilitation. In December, 2000 we participated in the Kinesio® Taping Instructors course. The positive results that occurred from taping our family, friends and co-workers eventually gave us the courage to tape the children we treat. We have been guided in our clinical experience in pediatrics to develop additional techniques as well as to refine the taping techniques for varied pediatric concerns. We have also combined other therapeutic interventions in conjunction with taping; such as splinting, compression bracing, and casting.

It is our hope that this book conveys treatment for children in a practical and understandable manner. This book is designed to describe the taping procedure by outlining specific taping techniques, step-by-step. The accompanying photographs help to clarify these procedures.

We also caution that Kinesio® Tex Tape application does carry some risk. We recommend taking a Kinesio® Taping course and collaborating with other professionals who have experience with the Kinesio® Taping applications.

While teaching throughout the country, we have met many talented pediatric therapists who have incorporated the Kinesio® Taping Method into their specialty areas. The excitement of taping pediatric clients has been overwhelming. Our hope is that clinical practitioners learn to enhance the management of the pediatric population based on sound clinical rationale and proper taping technique. We encourage clinicians to continue to develop diagnosis-specific taping techniques for the pediatric population and to share this with the Kinesio® Taping practitioners.

Lastly, we are grateful for the opportunity to learn and collaborate with our "sensei", Dr. Kase, in the development of this pediatric Kinesio® Taping book.

Trish Martin
Audrey Yasukawa

ACKNOWLEDGMENTS

We acknowledge the following people, who have been instrumental in the compilation and completion of this book:

Editors:
Nancy Dilger, Colleen Harper, Alice Marie Laverdiere, Carolyn Leitch, and Mary Saloka Morrison

Photographers:
Cel Jarvis
Marianne Mangan

The beautiful children who modeled for the book:
Austin, Celine, Daniel, Jamie, Julia, Kevin, Margaret, Maria, Meg, Megan, Mickey, Molly, Molly Mac, Rachael, Seamus, and Teresa

Kiyoko Simmons for her help during the early stages of this book
Tomoko Kase for her encouragement and support
John Jarvis for feedback from the field
Carol Salisbury and the staff of Kinesio® USA
Mike McDuffie from Kinesio® USA

Beverly Cusick for our initiation into the world of taping and the development of our knowledge base on biomechanical alignment.

We thank our families for allowing us to teach and to work on this special project.
Audrey thanks her husband Danny and son Miles Faith.
Trish thanks her husband Jimmy and children Jennifer, Jamie, Colleen and Molly.

GENERAL INTRODUCTION TO KINESIO® TAPING

by Kenzo Kase, DC, Founder

Some physicians and therapists who treat neuromuscular diseases liken the process of diagnosing nerve and muscle conditions to solving crimes. In law investigations, detectives and forensic scientists use DNA samples, fingerprints, and technology and science to determine the cause and relations of their cases. Neuromuscular therapists also use clues—namely presenting symptoms, medical histories, and physical examination results to pinpoint the culprit behind their patients' symptoms.

I look to the body as a whole, one muscle connecting to another, intertwined with connective tissue, ligament, fascia, and lymph functions. The Kinesio® Taping Method offers therapists a window into Advance Healing; to treat only the specific area or problem is to ignore the rest of the body. The Kinesio® Taping Method is a complete approach to healing; by taking a look at not only the problem area, but also those areas associated with the condition. This being said, the applications of Kinesio® Tape are endless in the pediatric field. It is in the area of strained muscles and weak joints that Kinesio® may be best known, but it is the technique's versatility that makes it most effective.

One problem therapists face is the child's lack of carryover from the weekly therapy session. With the use of the Kinesio® Taping Method, one can take the therapy home. The child is able to take the "hands" of the therapist out of the visit and utilize Kinesio® Tex Tape on a 24-hour basis. It is paramount that ongoing input be relayed to the child's neuromuscular system over multiple days to see qualitative results.

The objective of this book and the Kinesio® Taping Method is to offer the therapists a foundation of applications that will aid in the process of re-educating the conditions that affect such a wide variety of your patient population. Kinesio® Taping is proud to be involved in the aid and treatment of our pediatric population, and it is with your help we are able to do so. I would also like to give a special thanks to Audrey Yasukawa, OT, CKTI and Trish Martin, PT, CKTI -- without their hard work, foresight, and commitment to the Kinesio® Taping Method and their patients, this book would not be possible. It is through a healthy child that we have a healthy world. Through Kinesio® we can achieve both.

Fundamentals of Kinesio® Taping

Kinesio® Tex Tape is made of 100% cotton and has elastic properties. It is this property that allows Kinesio® Tex Tape to work with the soft tissue of the body versus restricting it. It is the elasticity that makes Kinesio® Tex Tape a good modality for the treatment of lymphoedema and chronic swelling.

Many of the Kinesio® Tapings applications may look similar. However the tapings can be for very different purposes. For example, a taping for muscle tightness may look like a taping for muscle weakness. How the tape is applied can determine how it works on the soft tissue. It is important to read the directions of each of the taping methods carefully before applying the tape. Applying the tape correctly can greatly enhance the therapeutic benefits.

PROPERTIES OF KINESIO® TEX TAPE

- Kinesio® Tex Tape is made of 100% cotton. It is free of Latex.
- The tape is applied to the backing paper with 10% available stretch.
- The tape can be stretched 40-60% from the resting length (with 60% being the maximal stretch of the tape).
- The adhesive on the tape is medical grade acrylic and is heat sensitive. Rubbing the tape after application allows the tape to adhere better on to the skin.
- Kinesio® Tex Tape is latex free.
- The thickness and weight of tape is approximately that of skin, also the elastic properties of the tape is similar to skin as well. Therefore most patients easily tolerate the tape.
- The tape is a one-way stretch tape. The tape stretches along the longitudinal axis only.
- The tape allows free movement and does not restrict like conventional athletic taping. However the tape can be used similarly to athletic tape if the tension used is greater than 75% of the resting length.
- Tape can be applied as the paper is being removed off the tape. Majority of the applications will be done with what is called "paper-off tension". This is the tension on the tape as the tape is being applied while removing the paper backing. This is approximately 10-15% of the available stretch in the tape.
- The elastic properties of the tape can provide support and help to reduce muscle fatigue.
- The tape can stimulate muscles to strengthen when weak.
- The tape can also help encourage a relaxing of soft tissue and improve lymphatic flow. This in turn reduces pain and swelling.
- Kinesio Tex Tape affects the skin, fascia, muscles, joints, lymphatic and circulatory systems.

GENERAL PRINCIPLES OF KINESIO® TAPING

1. The anchors and ends of the tape are applied with no tension.

2. The tape can be left on for 3-5 days. Skin cells slough off in approximately 3-5 days which makes tape easier to take off. Do not leave the tape on for any longer than this amount of time.

3. The skin needs to rest for at least 24 hours after a taping application. However you can tape a different body area so continuous therapeutic input to soft tissue is possible. It is important to assess the skin prior and after any taping application. Some patients may need longer than the 24 hour resting time.

4. The patient can shower and /or bathe with tape on. Do not use a hair dryer to dry the tape. This can cause the tape to adhere too aggressively to the skin. Use a towel to dab tape dry.

5. Be sure to remove the tape immediately and gently if there is any skin irritation and/or sensitivity. If there is a question on whether a patient has skin sensitivities to the tape, try a test piece (2-3 inches) of Kinesio® Tex Tape with no tension prior to any therapeutic taping application on to that area. Leave the tape on for 24 hours or unless the patient notices any skin irritation (visual or sensory). If any sensitivity is noted do not use Kinesio® Tex Tape on this patient.

6. The majority of taping typically stays within the 10-15% tension (paper-off) of available stretch for therapeutic applications. (Most skin irritation is due to too much tension being applied to the tape).

7. Apply the tape approximately 20-30 minutes prior to an activity that has exposure to heat or sweat such as in a sporting activity.

8. Application of the tape can be done over a slight amount of hair. However if there is too much body hair, the patient will not have enough tape to skin contact to be effective. Clipping or shaving the hair may be needed.

9. For best results, apply the Kinesio® Tex Tape to both the painful area and the cause of the pain.

STRETCH AND RECOIL PRINCIPLES OF THE KINESIO® TEX TAPE

1. Stretch the tape away from anchor (portion with no tension) and the tail (portion with tension) will recoil back to anchor.
2. In the case when there is an anchor on both ends, stretch both anchors away from the middle. The tape will recoil back to the middle.
3. To encourage shortening of muscle to facilitate, tape origin to insertion.
4. To encourage elongation of muscle to inhibit, tape insertion to origin.
5. Start the anchor in the direction you want the lymphatics to flow to. The tails will want to recoil back to the anchor, directing the lymphatics to flow toward the anchor.

PARTS OF KINESIO® TAPING APPLICATION

1. **Anchor:** The anchors are a portion of the tape that has no tension applied. It is typically the first 1-inch to 2-inch (2.5cm to 5cm). Majority of the time it is the starting end of the tape. However in some taping applications it can be at both ends, in the middle, or it is applied at the finishing ends. It is important to note that on some of the tapings with higher than typical tension levels 75-100% you need to increase the size of the anchors to help distribute the forces on the skin. This will help the patient tolerate the higher tensions better and reduce the risk of soft tissue problems.

2. **Tail:** The tail is the portion of the tape where tension is applied to the tape. This is the working part of the tape. This typically starts at the anchor and then goes to the end of the tape. It is the split in the tape for a "Y", "X", or fan.

3. **Ends:** The last part of the tape that is laid down with down with no tension.

4. **Base:** The tape beyond the anchor. It is the "I" tape between the anchor and the beginning of the tails in a "Y" or "X" cut, or between the anchor and the end of an "I" cut.

GLOSSARY OF KINESIO® TAPING

Therapeutic Zone: Tape over the target tissue.

Tension: The amount of stretch applied to the tape; specified as a %.

Paper-off Tension: 10-15%

Tissue Stretch: Elongation of the target tissue. This can be active or with manual assist.

Proximal: Attachment closest to midline of the body (origin).

Distal: Attachment furthest from the midline (insertion).

Facilitation: Stimulus to activate muscle.

Inhibition: Stimulus provided to relax muscle.

Therapeutic Direction: Direction of recoil of the applied Kinesio® Tex Tape toward the anchor.

SHAPES OF KINESIO® TEX TAPE CUTS

"I" Shaped Taping

"I' shaped tapes are cut Kinesio® Tex Tapes with rounded ends. "I" shaped tapes are used for muscle taping, correctional tapings, indurated tissue, and scar management.

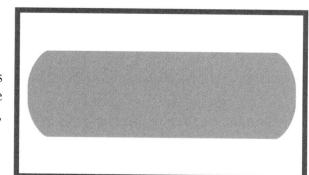

"Y" Shaped Taping

"Y" shaped tapes are Kinesio® Tex Tapes with one end that has a longitudinal cut in the middle of the tape. "Y" shaped tapes are used for muscle tapings, correctional tapings, indurated tissue, and scar taping.

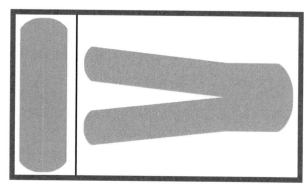

"X" Shaped Taping

"X" shaped tapes are Kinesio® Tex Tapes with both ends that have longitudinal cuts in the middle of the tape. "X" shaped tapes are used for muscle tapings, and correctional tapings.

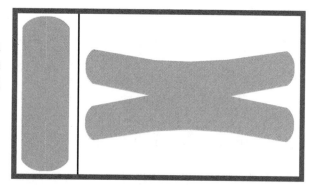

"Web" Shaped Taping

Web shaped tapes have 4-6 longitudinal strips in the middle of 2" wide Kinesio® Tex Tape and 6-8 longitudinal strips in the middle of 3" wide Kinesio® Tex Tape. This style of tape is used for correctional tapings, and indurated tissue.

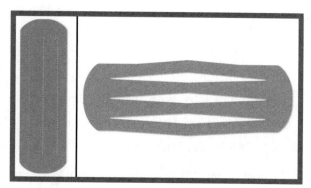

"Fan" Shaped Taping

Fan shaped tapes have 4-6 longitudinal strips on one end of 2" wide Kinesio® Tex Tape and 6-8 longitudinal strips on one end of 3" wide Kinesio® Tex Tape. Fan taping is used for correctional taping, and indurated tissue.

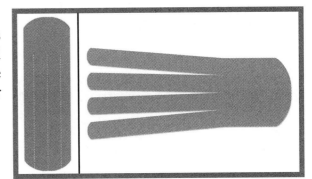

"X" Shaped Taping with "Donut" Hole

"X" shaped taping with hole in the middle of Kinesio® Tex Tape with both ends that have longitudinal cuts in the middle of the tape. This tape also has a hole cut in the middle of the tape. "X" shaped tapes are used for correctional tapings and indurated tissue.

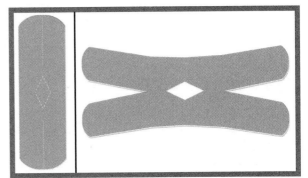

Basket Cut (Closed and Open Ended)

Closed ended basket cut has alternating 3 strips and 4 strips cut in a 2" wide Kinesio® Tex Tape and 5 strips and 6 strips in a 3" wide Kinesio® Tex Tape. Closed-ended basket cut tape is use for correctional taping, and indurated tissue.

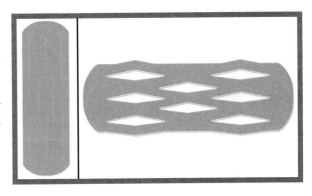

Open ended basket cut has alternating 3 strips and 4 strips cut in a 2" wide Kinesio® Tex Tape and 5 strips and 6 strips in a 3" wide Kinesio® Tex Tape. Open-ended basket cut tape is use for correction taping, and indurated tissue.

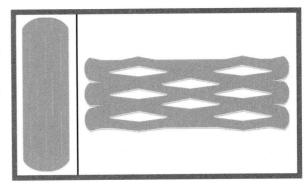

TAPE APPLICATION

- Prior to tape application, make sure the skin is clean. The skin should be free of oils and be dry. A spray adherent or skin preparation wipe can be used on skin that has difficulty keeping the tape adhered. Be careful for pediatric and any other patient with sensitive skin.
- Typically the joint is moved through a full active or passive range of motion to provide a stretch on the tissue. But in cases when more input is needed alternate position may be recommended.
- Lightly rubbing the tape activates the medical grade acrylic adhesive. This encourages the tape to adhere quickly to the skin.
- Avoid using hot packs or a heating source on Kinesio® Tex Tape.

REMOVAL OF TAPE

- It is more comfortable to gently remove the tape in the direction of hair growth.
- The tape can be gently rolled off the skin slowly using the base of one hand. Use the fingers of the other hand to support the skin to reduce discomfort as the tape is being removed.
- -Or- Support the skin with the fingers of one hand while the tape is being slowly and gently removed with the other hand.
- Tape may be removed while showering or in bath.

KINESIO® TAPING TENSION PERCENTAGES GUIDELINES:
(Percentage of Available Stretch in the Tape)

None	Very Light or Paper-Off	Light	Moderate	Severe	Full
0%	10-15%	15-25%	25-50%	50-75%	75-100%

General Introduction

PROPERTIES OF KINESIO® TEX TAPE

Kinesio® Tex Tape has been modified, since its creation, to mimic the qualities of the skin. In understanding the overlying concepts of the Kinesio® Taping Method, it is best to think of the basic and corrective techniques as the application/placement of your hands onto the patient. Keeping the concept of the tape replicating the placement of your hand on the patient, in combination with the tape mimicking the qualities of the skin, will assist you as you try to learn the Kinesio® Taping Method.

Kinesio® Tex Tape has been designed to allow for a longitudinal stretch of 40-60 % of its resting length. This degree of stretch approximates the elastic qualities of the human skin. The tape is not designed to stretch horizontally. The Kinesio® Tex Tape is applied to the paper substrate with approximately 10-15% of available tension. The average roll of Kinesio® Tex Tape can stretch 40-60% from its resting length. The elastic qualities of the Kinesio® Tex Tape are effective for 3-5 days before the elastic polymer diminishes.

The thickness of the Kinesio® Tex Tape is approximately the same as the epidermis of the skin. This was intended to limit the body's perception of weight and avoid sensory stimuli when properly applied. After approximately 10 minutes, the patient will generally not perceive there is tape on their skin.

The Kinesio® Tex Tape is comprised of a polymer elastic strand wrapped by 100% cotton fibers. The cotton fibers allow for evaporation of body moisture and allow for quick drying.

There is no latex in the tape. The adhesive is 100% acrylic and is heat activated. The skin must be free of oils and moisture prior to application. The acrylic adhesive becomes more adherent the longer the Kinesio® Tex Tape is worn. The acrylic adhesive is applied in a wave-like pattern to mimic the qualities of the fingerprint on the fingertip. This not only assists in the lifting of the skin, but also allows for zones in which moisture can escape.

Upon removal of the Kinesio® Tex Tape, there will be no glue residue remaining. This normally allows for multiple taping technique applications without skin irritation. If the patient has sensitive skin, it is recommended that the practitioner apply a small strip of tape and evaluate the patient's reaction prior to full use.

The combination of the stretch capabilities, thickness, and adhesion allow the Kinesio® Tex Tape to approximate the qualities of the skin. The design of the Kinesio® Tex Tape, in combination with the unique application technique, create the Kinesio® Taping Method.

BASIC APPLICATION ESSENTIALS

The success of the Kinesio® Taping Method is dependent upon two factors. One, proper evaluation of the patient's condition to allow for application of Kinesio® Tex Tape on the proper tissue. Two, proper application of the Kinesio® Taping Technique. When the two are combined, an effective treatment modality is available to the practitioner. Early in the learning process, many practitioners believe they can utilize the method with little practice. Generally, this is true. However, success is limited by the practitioner's ability to evaluate the patient's condition and the possibility of mistakes in tape application. As stated previously, it is recommended that for the Kinesio® Taping Method a tape with elasticity from 35-40 % be used. Using a tape which has a different adhesive, is thicker, does not breath, and has different elastic qualities will not produce the same results.

Primarily, the practitioner needs to "unlearn" tape application methods which have been previously learned. During conventional athletic taping, proper application requires using all of the available stretch. The concept is that by taking all of the stretch out of the tape, it will limit or assist a motion and provide for protection from injury/re-injury.

With the Kinesio® Taping Method, the practitioner needs to begin to conceptualize that the Kinesio® Tex Tape will assist the body's return to normal function through the application of the tape onto the skin. The primary effect of tape application is generally superficial and by applying the Kinesio® Tex Tape with excess tension it's effectiveness will be limited.

SKIN PREPARATION

The skin should be free of oils and lotions and should be cleaned prior to tape application. Anything that limits the acrylic adhesive's ability to adhere to the skin will limit both effectiveness and length of application.

For a limited number of patients, body hair may limit adhesion. If the degree of body hair limits adhesion then the practitioner may need to shave or clip the area to be treated. If applying tape in an area of moisture, the water resistant product may be preferable.

REMOVAL OF TAPE FROM PAPER BACKING

To smoothly remove the paper backing, hold the tape vertically, place your index finger on the top edge of the tape. Then by pulling back or flexing your index finger towards your body, the tape will peel from its backing.

Any contact with the acrylic adhesive will diminish its adhesive abilities. Try to touch the adhesive as little as possible.

When removing the Kinesio® Tex Tape from the paper backing, only remove the amount required to begin the base application. Once base application is completed, the practitioner may want to peel the remaining paper backing away. When doing this, be careful to remove the backing while remembering that 10-15% of available tension is applied to the tape during manufacturing.

Two other common methods are used to remove the tape from the paper backing. One, tear paper backing just below the base of a Y cut, leaving the paper backing on the tails. As each tail is applied, the Kinesio® Tex Tape can be removed from the paper substrate using the paper off tension (10-15%). Two, remove the paper backing from the tails and lightly have the Kinesio® Tex Tape come into contact with the skin. Do not rub the Kinesio® Tex Tape as this will initiate glue adhesion. As the Kinesio® Tex Tape contacts the skin, it will grab the skin and be held in place.

If care is not taken in removing the paper backing from the Kinesio® Tex Tape, it may roll back and adhere to itself, making application difficult.

SELECTION OF KINESIO® STRIP TYPE

Kinesio® strip can be applied in the shape of a "Y", "I", "X", "Fan", "Web", and "Donut". The shape selected depends upon the size of the affected muscle and desired treatment effect.

The "Y" technique is the most common method of application. It is used for surrounding a muscle to either facilitate or inhibit muscle stimuli. The basic principle of therapeutic taping for weakened muscles is to wrap the tape around the affected muscle. This is accomplished by using the "Y" strip. The "Y" strip should be approximately two inches longer than the muscle, measured from Origin to Insertion.

The "I" strip can be used in place of the "Y" strip for an acutely injured muscle. The primary purpose of tape application following acute injury is to limit edema and pain.

The "X" strip is used when a muscle's Origin and Insertion may change depending upon the movement pattern of the joint (e.g.: Rhomboid).

The "Fan" strip is used for lymphatic drainage which is an advanced concept.

The "Web" is a modified fan cut. Both base ends are left intact, with the strips being cut in the mid section of the Kinesio® strip.

The "Donut" cut is primarily used for edema in a focal or sport-specific area. A series of two or three overlapping strips are applied with the center removed from the Kinesio® Tex Tape. The center cut out, or "donut hole" is placed directly over the area to be treated.

With any of the five strip types, it is helpful to round the ends of the tape prior to application. The rounding helps prevent the square edges from catching and may increase the length of tape application.

ANCHOR APPLICATION

Following proper evaluation of the tissues involved, the practitioner determines to which basic muscles the Kinesio® Taping Method should be applied. Begin by placing the anchor of the Kinesio® strip approximately 2 inches below the origin (proximal part) or two inches above the insertion (distal part) of the muscle. (To determine origin or insertion of desired muscle, the practitioner may use manual muscle testing to determine application start and /or ending point).Place the anchor in as close to an anatomical position as possible. Make sure to rub the anchor prior to completing the taping technique. The base of the Kinesio® strip is always started and ended with no tension in order to minimize discomfort from tape application.

TISSUE STRETCH

For all basic application techniques, the muscle/tissue to be treated should be put in a stretched position in combination with the stretch capabilities of the Kinesio® Tex Tape, will create convolutions as the skin is lifted. Skin convolutions may be present following the basic application or may appear during normal joint motion. It is believed that even if convolutions are not present, they are occurring. The convolutions aid in the normal flow of blood and lymphatic fluids.

TAPE STRETCH/TENSION

The elastic qualities of the Kinesio® Tex Tape are designed for 40-60% stretch. When applying the Kinesio® Taping Method, it is important to apply the Kinesio® strip with the correct degree of tension. If too much tension is applied, the effects are diminished. It is better not to have enough tension than too much. The proper tension application is one of the most critical factors in the application's success. The terms "stretch" or "tension" are used interchangeably. In each taping method, including basic, corrective techniques, and clinical conditions, the tension during tape application is critical.

Tape stretch tensions are listed as a percentage and descriptively. Percentages are listed as the percentage of stretch to be applied based upon 100% of the available tension. For example, 15-25%. The meaning of this is 15-25% of the available stretch, with 100 % being the maximum stretch.

If you start with a 10-inch strip of Kinesio® Tex Tape, and you stretch it to it's maximum available tension (40-60% of overall length), it would be 14 inches long. During application, if the technique requires 25% of the available tension, this would actually be 25% of the total available or 1 inch for a total length of 11 inches.

Tensions are also listed descriptively by terms which should convey the amount of tension desired.

Descriptions used are:

none -- (0%)

very light or paper off -- (10-15%)

light -- (15-25%)

moderate -- (25-50%)

severe -- (50-75%)

full -- (75-100%)

TAPE DIRECTION

There are two basic application directions for treatment of muscles. For acutely over-used or stretched muscles, the tape is applied from INSERTION to ORIGIN (DISTAL to PROXIMAL) to inhibit muscle function. For chronically weak muscles or where increased contraction is desired, the tape is applied from ORIGIN to INSERTION (PROXIMAL to DISTAL) to facilitate muscle function.

INSERTION to ORIGIN application tape stretch/tension is very light or light, 15-25% of available tension. Using the preferred Kinesio® Tex Tape, this would simply require applying the tape by placing it on the muscle as it comes off of the paper backing (paper off tension). Remember that the Kinesio® Tex Tape is applied to the paper

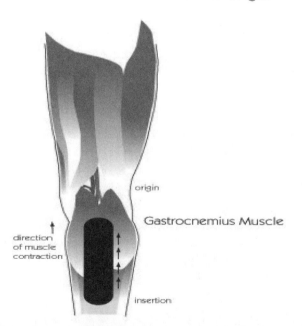

Insertion to Origin

origin

Gastrocnemius Muscle

direction of muscle contraction

insertion

backing with approximately 10-15% of available stretch/tension. With taping from insertion to origin, it is important to remember that "less is better". Applying too much tension decreases desired results instead of enhancing them. If, following tape application, the practitioner can see any depression in the skin, the tape is applied with too much tension/stretch.

ORIGIN to INSERTION application tension is light to moderate, 25-50% of available tension. When applying the Kinesio® Tex Tape with proper application technique for ORIGIN to INSERTION, the practitioner should be able to see slight separation of the elastic fibers in the Kinesio® Tex Tape.

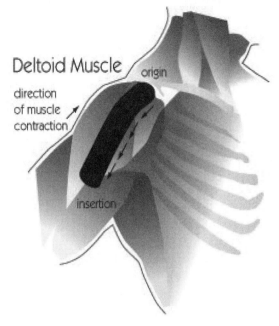

Origin to Insertion

"Y" STRIP APPLICATION

With the skin properly prepared, anchor is applied with no tension, and muscle/tissue on a stretch, it is now time to apply the Kinesio® strip. Surround the muscle to be taped by laying down one of the two tails of the "Y" strip. Tension is applied evenly along the tail. As the tape is being laid down, follow behind with a thumb or finger and rub the tape onto the skin to initiate glue adhesion. When the tail of the tape is approximately one to two inches from the end, stop tension and lay the end down with no tension. Again, rub the applied tape strip to initiate glue adhesion prior to moving the muscle from its current stretched position.

Where appropriate, place the muscle in a second stretched position to apply the second tail of the "Y" strip. Follow the above description for the second tail.

A three strip "Y" technique may also be selected. The third tail is applied directly over the muscle belly.

Once the basic application is complete, it is important to instruct the patient about a few areas of concern. The tape needs approximately 20 minutes to gain full adhesive strength. Exercise or activities which may initiate perspiration should not occur during this period. The tape can be worn for 3-4 days, and bathing or swimming is allowed. It is important to pat the tape dry and not use any type of heat device to dry the tape. The patient also needs to be comfortable with wearing the tape in a public setting.

"I" STRIP APPLICATION

The application of the "I" technique follows the same basic principles as the "Y" technique in the Peds book for this entire section. Instead of surrounding the muscle belly, the Kinesio® strip is applied directly over the area of injury or pain. This technique has been found to be most effective following acute injuries to the muscle. Immediately following a muscle injury, the "I" technique should be applied. Then, after the acute injury phase, the practitioner may find increased results by switching to the "Y" technique.

"X" STRIP APPLICATION

The "X" application follows the same principles as the "Y" and "I" taping techniques. The length of the "X" strip is measured with the muscle on a stretch. This is important, since an "X" technique is generally used for a muscle which crosses two joints and when it is maximally stretched it may greatly increase in length. The stretch is added to the middle 1/3 of the "X" strip, placed over the muscle belly, and the tails are laid down with no tension. The center may also be laid down with no tension, and tension applied to the tails.

"FAN" STRIP APPLICATION

The Fan Strip is applied with the muscle in a stretched position. For lymphatic correction, none to very light, 0-15%, of available tension is added to the Kinesio® Tex Tape Fan Strip tails (4-8). The Fan Strip tails are laid over the area of edema or swelling, with the base located in the area of a lymphatic duct. For a more complete description, see Lymphatic Corrective Technique.

"WEB" STRIP APPLICATION

Cut the middle of the Kinesio® Tape into 4-8 strips. The Kinesio® Tex Tape is cut allowing for each end to remain uncut. Place patient in as much range of motion as the joint will allow. Apply one base, remove the web strips, add very light 0-15% of available tension and apply the second base. For a more complete description, see Space Corrective Technique.

"DONUT" STRIP APPLICATION

Begin by cutting a hole in the center of an approximately 6 inches Kinesio® I strip. Cut approximately 2 inches of each end into two or three tails. Place patient in as much range of motion as the joint will allow. Apply light to moderate, 25-50%, of available tension to the Kinesio® strip, and place the hole directly over the area of desired space. If more than one strip is applied, use light tension. For a more complete description, see Space Corrective Technique.

TAPE REMOVAL

After several days the acrylic adhesive will have become quite strong. During the first few days, if an edge of the tape has begun to lift, it can be trimmed. To remove the tape from the patient it is generally much easier to do when they have bathed or the tape is moist. It is best to remove from the top down. This will be in the direction of the body hair and should limit discomfort. Lift the tape from the skin, applying tension between the skin and the tape, then push the skin away from the tape rather than pulling the tape away from the skin.

If the "grip and rip" method is used, an irritation, pain and erythema may result. The application of mineral oil or milk of magnesia to the Kinesio® Tex Tape has assisted in tape removal.

POSSIBLE LIMITATIONS OF KINESIO® TAPING METHOD

A limited number of patients may have excessive body hair and may require shaving or clipping. A limited number of patients may not allow the application of the Kinesio® Taping Method due to their resistance to shaving.

Approximately 20-30 minutes is required for the glue to become fully activated before the patient can become physically active. If activity occurs prior to this time, the tape may come off.

If Kinesio® Tex Tape is applied during physical activity, an extra adhesive may be needed to prepare the skin. Several commercially produced spray adherents are available. Once a spray adherent is used, the removal of the Kinesio® Tex Tape will be difficult. Commonly available tape adherent glue removers will not affect the adhesive glue since it is not rubber based as most athletic tapes.

The patient may be unwilling or may misunderstand the three to four day application of the technique. The patient must be aware that the tape is to remain on for several days and can be worn while bathing or swimming. The tape does not have to be removed if it has become wet, only towel off excessive moisture and allow to air dry.

INITIAL DIFFICULTIES IN APPLICATION

The practitioner will need to "unlearn" previous training for use of athletic tapes. Pulling and using full stretch will diminish the effectiveness of this technique. One must begin to think differently about the possible therapeutic use of tape beyond simply assisting or limiting a movement.

A proper muscle evaluation is required to ensure the correct muscle is selected for treatment. If, following the initial Kinesio® Taping Technique application, the patient's results were not as effective as hoped, the practitioner may want to reevaluate the patient. If the involved muscle was not properly taped, or an inappropriate corrective technique was applied, patient success may be limited.

SIZES AND TYPES OF KINESIO® TEX TAPE

There are several sizes of the Kinesio® Tex Tape available. Primarily a practitioner will use the 2 inches (5 cm) by 5.4 yards (5 meters) size. The 2 inch Kinesio® Tex Tape size can also be purchased in a 34.5 yard (31m) clinic roll for easier usage.

Also available is a 3 inch (7.5 cm) by 5.4 yards (5 meters) roll. This may be required on larger individuals or athletes. The 1 inch (2.5 cm) by 5.4 yard (5 meters) roll may be used for finger or neurological taping.

The Kinesio® Tex Tape is available in red, blue, and black in addition to the beige or natural color. The red is a darker color on the light spectrum and will absorb more light, slightly increasing the temperature under the Kinesio® Tex Tape strip. The blue is a lighter color on the light spectrum and will reflect more light, slightly decreasing the temperature under the Kinesio® Tex Tape Strip. There are no differences in the manufacture of the tape except the change in the dye color required for a color difference.

If the practitioner determines an increase in temperature is appropriate in the injury site, the red Kinesio® Tex Tape could be selected. If the practitioner believes that a reduction in tissue temperature is required, such as in tendonitis, the blue Kinesio® Tex Tape could be selected. Patients may have a preference for a color, and this may affect their perception of the effectiveness of the treatment.

ADVANCED APPLICATION ESSENTIALS

When applying the corrective techniques, there are a few essentials to a successful treatment for the patient. The practitioner must always follow the basic essentials of tape application when using a basic Kinesio® Taping Technique muscle application. Without properly applying the basic muscle application technique, the success of the corrective technique application may be limited. Proper skin preparation, removal of tape from paper backing, selection of tape width, tissue stretch, tape tension, direction of tape application, glue activation, and tape removal are all important in the overall successful treatment of the patient.

When applying more than one layer of the Kinesio® Tex Tape, the practitioner should first apply the Kinesio® strip which will provide the primary therapeutic effect desired. As successive layers of Kinesio® Tex Tape are applied, their effect on the sensory receptors may create interference instead of clear, specific stimuli.

If the primary therapeutic goal is pain reduction, the practitioner may use a basic muscle technique from insertion to origin, along with a space correction or lymphatic correction. The practitioner may determine that the application of the lymphatic correction should be applied for the first 24-72 hours, then apply a space correction technique. After 72 hours, application of the basic muscle technique with a mechanical correction may be appropriate.

The best outcomes generally come from a "less is better" approach. Fewer layers of tape, less tension, and moderate inward pressure are examples of subtle changes transmitted from the Kinesio® Tex Tape to the superficial layers of the tissue.

During initial applications of the Kinesio® Taping Method, the patient should tell the practitioner if he or she is feeling the effects. In this instance the tape application can be modified for possible improvement in results. If the patient returns and believes the tape application exacerbated the symptoms, the ability of the practitioner to successfully treat the patient is limited.

The descriptions provided for the clinical conditions are not intended to be the only method of tape application for any condition. They are intended to be guides. The techniques described have been found in clinical practice to show results after repeated applications with many patients. Every patient presents his own specific symptoms, and the practitioner, through knowledge and experience, will determine the most appropriate course of treatment.

Introduction to Corrective Techniques

The Corrective Application Techniques are a continuation in the development of the Kinesio® Taping Method. Since 1973, when the original concept of the Kinesio® Taping Method was begun, the technique has continued to evolve. This continuing development has added not only to the theoretical application, but also to the practical application, of the technique. Kinesio® Taping Practitioners have developed their skills both by learning during seminars and via practical application. The Corrective Techniques have been formalized to help the Kinesio® Taping Practitioner gain application and theoretical knowledge in a more systematic fashion. During Kinesio® Taping seminars, practitioners desiring to learn the Kinesio® Taping Method have traditionally followed a 2 day basic Kinesio® Taping course. The introduction to the Kinesio® Taping Method reviews the basic concepts of the technique; followed by the lab experience of the basic application. The therapists are encouraged to practice and apply the taping techniques on their patients. After clinical practice and refinement of the taping techniques, therapists can further develop their skills and problem solving abilities through attending advanced Kinesio® Taping courses.

Difficulties have arisen when a practitioner has completed a course and been introduced to clinical applications without receiving advanced training (Corrective Techniques). Many practitioners have thought that each clinical application was unique. This required the practitioner, in their mind, to learn each clinical application separately with little or no interconnection. In reality, this is not true.

The clinical application of the Kinesio® Taping Method is the systematic application of several elements of the Kinesio® Taping Technique with each element having a specific function. The practitioner initially evaluates the patient's condition, determines which muscles are involved and initiates treatment to those muscles involved (basic concepts and application). Once the involved muscles are taped, the practitioner then needs to apply a clinical corrective technique to assist the body in correcting the condition.

There are 6 current Corrective Techniques: mechanical, fascia, space, ligament/tendon, functional, and lymphatic. The application methods of several of the Corrective Techniques overlap. The Kinesio® Taping Practitioner determines the proper application following his/her evaluation.

CORRECTIVE APPLICATION TECHNIQUES

When using corrective techniques, the anchors must be longer to dissipate the tension on the skin.

Mechanical Correction "Recoiling" – utilizes the stretching qualities of the Kinesio® Tex Tape with inward pressure to provide for positional stimuli through the skin. The degree of stimulation is determined by the percentage of stretch applied to the tape during application, combined with the degree of inward pressure. Three techniques used are: 1) using the base of the "Y" to provide tension, 2) using the tails of the "Y" to provide tension, and 3) using the tension in the center of an I strip. Mechanical correction generally uses moderate to severe 25-75% of available tension. The practitioner may select to use full tension, if appropriate.

Fascia Correction "Holding" – to create and/or gather fascia in order to align the tissue in the desired position. The tension in the Kinesio® Tex Tape is used to either hold or assist the fascia in the desired position. Two techniques are used: 1) manually positioning fascia then using tape to hold in place, 2) creating tension by "oscillating" the tape and creating movement of the fascia. Fascia correction, generally, uses light to moderate 15-50% of available tension.

Space Correction "Lifting" – to create more space directly above the area of pain, inflammation, swelling, or edema. The increased space is believed to reduce pressure by lifting the skin. Three techniques are used: 1) manually gather tissue into desired position and use tension of Kinesio® Tex Tape to hold
the position of the tissue, 2) utilize fascia technique of "oscillation", 3) use elastic qualities of Kinesio® Tex Tape to pull and hold connective tissue in desired area.
Space correction generally uses light to moderate, or 25-50% of available tension.

Ligament/Tendon Correction "Pressure" – to create increased stimulation over the area of the ligament and/or tendon, resulting in increased stimulation of the mechanoreceptors. The stimulus is believed to be perceived as proprioceptive, simulating more normal tissue. Ligament technique: Kinesio® Tex Tape is placed over the ligament with moderate to severe, or 50-75% of available tension. Tendon technique: tape over tendon is applied with moderate to severe, or 25-75+% of available tension.
For both techniques the practitioner may apply full, or 100% of available tension.

Functional Correction "Spring" – used when the practitioner desires a sensory stimulation to either assist or limit a motion. The Kinesio® Tex Tape is applied to the skin with moderate to full, or 50-75+% of available tension during active movement. The increased mechanoreceptor stimuli are believed to act as a pre-load during end of motion positions.

Lymphatic Correction "Channeling" – used to create areas of decreased pressure under the Kinesio® Tex Tape that act as channels to direct the exudate to the nearest lymph duct. Tape is applied with the base near the lymph node to which the exudate is to be directed, and the remaining tape is applied in a fan-like pattern with none to very light, or 10-25% of available tension.

The desired outcome is that, following a course in the Corrective Techniques, the practitioner will be able to select the technique appropriate for their patient's condition, and not be limited to only those specific applications they have seen in a photo or demonstrated in a seminar.
The practitioner should recognize that for each clinical condition they may use a series of Corrective Techniques depending on the patient's condition and the therapeutic goal of the practitioner. Pain reduction may be the first therapeutic goal, and application of a space or lymphatic correction may be selected. After pain has decreased, a mechanical correction or fascia correction might be selected. The Corrective Technique allows the practitioner the opportunity to design a course of treatment for each patient based upon the patient's needs and not a predetermined formula.

MECHANICAL CORRECTION

The Mechanical Correction should be thought of as positional in nature and not as an attempt to keep the tissue or joint in a fixed position. This technique uses the properties of the Kinesio® Tex Tape, through the application of moderate to severe tension, to provide a stimulus perceived by the mechanoreceptors. The degree of stimulation is determined by the combination of appropriate tension and inward pressure that provides stimulus to deeper tissue. You, as a practitioner, will need to adjust your application technique to the needs of the patient.

This technique can be used to assist in the positioning of muscle, fascia tissue, or joint to stimulate a sensation which results in the body's adaptation to the stimulus. Functional support can be maintained without losing active range of motion or inhibiting circulation. The Mechanical Correction can be used to either position the tissue in the desired position, provide stimulus in which the body will adjust position to minimize the created tension, or provide a "blocking" action of joint or tissue movement.

There are two methods used to place the tissue in the desired position: one, use of a manual technique, and, two, use of the elastic qualities of the Kinesio® Tex Tape. If using a manual therapy to provide positioning, first place the tissue in the correct or desired position, using techniques such as joint positioning or myofascial release, before applying the taping technique. When using the elastic qualities of the Kinesio® Tex Tape to provide correct positioning, tension can either be applied using the base of the Y (with the tails being used to dissipate the tension) or the tails (base of the Y is applied with no tension and the tails are stretched maximally with no tension on the ends).

A third method uses tension in the middle of the Kinesio® strip with inward pressure to create a "blocking" action. The approximately 6-8 inches long Kinesio® I strip is applied with moderate to full tension applied to the middle of the strip. The Kinesio® strip is then applied directly over the joint, or tissue with inward pressure. The desired effect is limited movement of the joint or tissue.

When selecting either method, manual or elastic qualities of the Kinesio® Tex Tape, the intent of the tape is to use the "recoil" effect of the elastic polymer. The tape application is completed so that when the tape "recoils" back to its original position it creates tension upon the skin which creates sensory stimuli. The practitioner can either use the stimulus effect of the elastic qualities of the tape to create a corrective reaction or position the tissue without movement.

The recoil effect of the Kinesio® Tex Tape is in effect up to approximately 50% of available tension. After applying more than 50% of available tension, the recoil effect is minimized due to the inability of the elastic polymer to recoil.

The application of inward pressure provides for a deeper stimulus to mechanoreceptors affecting deeper layers of tissue. The combination of high tension and inward pressure is the primary component of the mechanical corrective technique.

MECHANICAL CORRECTION APPLICATION TECHNIQUES
APPLICATION OF Y TECHNIQUE, TENSION ON TAILS
(LOW LEVEL STIMULUS)

Application of "Y" Technique with tension on tails of "Y": This technique uses the "recoil" effect of the elastic qualities of the tape to position the tissue in the direction of the base of the Kinesio® strip. The amount of stretch applied to the Kinesio® strip and degree of inward pressure determine the depth and perception of skin movement. By using tension in the tails, the practitioner is applying a subtle stimulus.

Anchor the tape with no tension at the beginning. Hold base of "Y" to beginning of tails to not create any tension to the anchor or base.

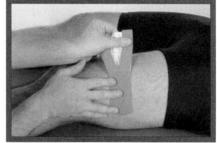

Apply the tails with moderate to severe tension, 50-75% of available. More tension can be applied over tendon or ligament. Tension is applied both in the longitudinal direction and with downward/inward pressure.

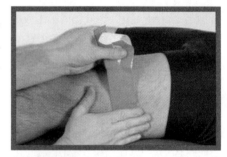

When the desired tension has been applied, slide the hand which is holding the base of the "Y" tails up to the point of end tension. Leave approximately a one-inch length of tape at end.

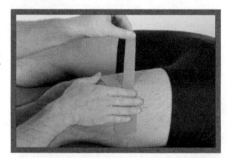

Lay down the final approximately 1 inch of remaining tape tails (ends) with no tension. Where appropriate, take joint through full range of motion prior to laying down ends.

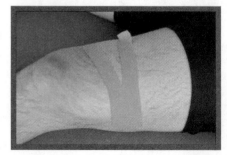

MECHANICAL CORRECTION APPLICATION TECHNIQUES
APPLICATION OF Y TECHNIQUE, WITH TENSION ON BASE
(MODERATE LEVEL STIMULUS)

Application of "Y" Technique with tension on base of "Y": This technique uses the base of the "Y" cut to apply tension to the skin. The amount of stretch applied to the Kinesio® strip and the degree of inward pressure determine the depth and perception of skin movement.

Anchor the tape with no tension at the beginning. Hold base of tape to not create any tension.

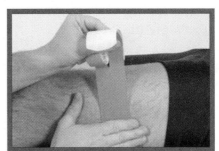

Apply moderate to severe, 50-75%, tension when applying the base of the "Y" strip over the tendon or the ligament. Tendon is applied both in the longitudinal direction and with downward/inward pressure. Prior to tape application, the practitioner may want to place the patient's joint in a position which may either stimulate or limit motion.

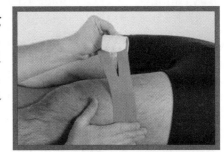

When the desired tension has been applied, slide the hand which is holding the base of the "Y" up to the point of end tension.

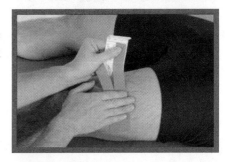

Lay down the tails of the "Y" with no tension as the patient moves through a full range of motion. The tails should be splayed out to dissipate the tension created over as large an area as possible.

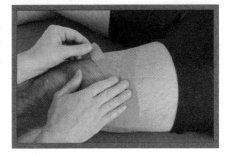

MECHANICAL CORRECTION APPLICATION TECHNIQUES
APPLICATION OF I TECHNIQUE, WITH TENSION IN THE CENTER OF THE TAPE
(HIGH LEVEL STIMULUS)

Application of "I" Technique with tension in the middle of Kinesio® strip: This technique uses the application of tension in the middle of the Kinesio® "I" strip and inward pressure to provide a "blocking" of movement. The amount of tension and inward pressure determine the degree of "blocking".

Fold the Kinesio® "I" strip in the center and tear the backing, fold back the edges. Begin by placing the center of the Kinesio® "I" strip, of approximately 6-8 inches in length, directly over the tissue to be treated (target tissue). Apply moderate to severe tension, 50-75% of available, to the middle of the strip. Place the Kinesio® strip over the treatment area with tension and downward/inward pressure. Use the Kinesio® strip to create a "block" to limit movement of a joint or tissue.

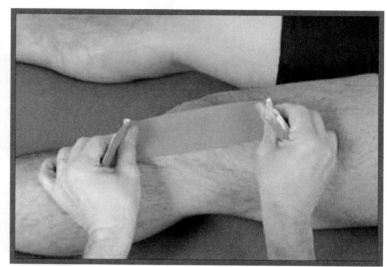

Have the patient move into a position which places the joint or tissue being treated in a stretched position. Lay down the ends of the Kinesio® "I" strip with no tension to dissipate the force added.

The application shown has approximately 1/2 of the Kinesio® "I" strip over the lateral border of the patella to limit lateral tracking.

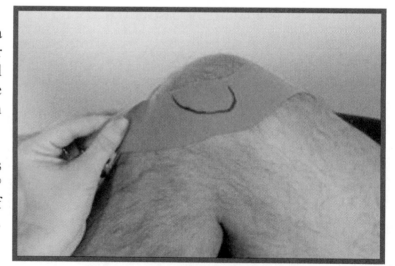

FASCIA CORRECTION

The fascia correction is applied to create and gather fascia tissue in order to position it in a desired alignment. Tape is applied to hold or assist fascia from unwinding to the unwanted position. This technique is intended to gently break down limitations of fascia movement via skin movement and elastic qualities of the Kinesio® Tex Tape.

Fascia is an interconnecting matrix that connects tissues from one layer to the next and within the same layer. It is like a 3-dimensional spiderweb which lies between each layer of tissue, and any acute or chronic inflammation there impairs the ability of the tissue to move.

The fascia technique is applied in two different application methods. First, one may use the elastic qualities of the Kinesio® Tex Tape to reposition the fascia or to limit its movement. Second, one may use the Kinesio® Tex Tape to hold the fascia in a desired position or limit its movement following application of a myofascial manual therapy technique.

The proper application technique for using the Kinesio® Tex Tape to hold a manual therapy technique is similar to the mechanical technique previously described. Following the manual therapy technique, the fascia is held in the desired position with one hand. The Kinesio® strip cut in a "Y" pattern is then applied to hold the tissue in the desired position. The specific difference between a fascia correction and a mechanical correction is the use of inward pressure. Inward pressure is only applied when the practitioner desires a deeper effect. Generally the fascia correction is applied with little or no inward pressure.

The proper application technique for using the elastic qualities of the Kinesio® Tex Tape involves the "oscillation" of the Kinesio® strip. Apply the base of the Y strip 1/2 to 1 inch below the area to be treated. The base is held to limit tension, and the practitioner "oscillates" or vibrates the tape in a longitudinal direction during application. The "oscillation" or vibration is gentle and may include a slight inward pressure if the effects are felt to be required in deeper tissues. This is felt to limit the "recoil" effect of the tape returning to its original position towards the base.

FASCIA CORRECTION APPLICATION TECHNIQUE
USE OF FASCIA CORRECTION TECHNIQUE TO REPOSITION FASCIA, TENSION ON THE BASE

Use of fascia Correction Technique to reposition fascia, with tension on the base: In this technique, the practitioner uses the elastic qualities of the Kinesio® Tex Tape to simulate a manual therapy technique. The elastic qualities of the Kinesio® Tex Tape will be applied using an "oscillating" motion in an attempt to reduce tension and adhesions between and within layers of the fascia. This technique may not be as effective as using a manual technique; however, if the practitioner is not skilled in a manual technique this may still allow an option for treatment.

Anchor the Kinesio® "Y" strip approximately 1/2 to 1 inch below the area of fascia to be treated, with no tension.

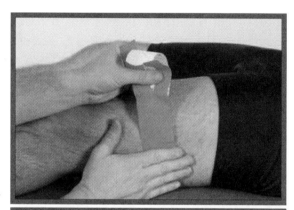

Apply light to moderate tension, (15-50% of available) to the tape in the direction fascia correction is desired. Hold the anchor with one hand to minimize excess tension on the anchor. The anchor of the "Y" strip should be "oscillated" in the longitudinal direction. Minimal inward pressure should also be applied as the tape is being laid down. The inward pressure is not specifically intended to deepen the effect of the tape, but is only used to apply the Kinesio® Tex Tape during application; its function is to reduce the "recoil" effect of the Kinesio® Tex Tape.

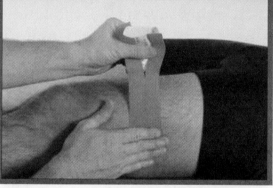

Lay down the tails of the Kinesio® "Y" strip with no tension.
This technique can also be used to pull the fascia in the opposite direction. If the practitioner desires to move the fascia "away from" an area, the elastic qualities of the Kinesio® Tex Tape can be used to accomplish this goal.

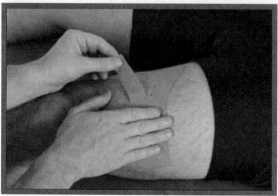

FASCIA CORRECTION APPLICATION TECHNIQUE
MANUAL FASCIA WINDING OR MYOFASCIAL RELEASE, TENSION ON BASE.

Use of manual fascia winding or myofascial release technique: Following the application of a manual therapy technique, position the fascia in the desired position prior to tape application. This technique can be used to either hold fascia in desired position or limit the movement of fascia into an unwanted position. Use the Kinesio® strip to hold the corrective positioning of the fascia.

Use a manual technique to collect or correct fascia and soft tissue as appropriate

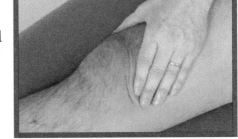

Anchor the tape slightly above or below soft tissue which has been gathered. Placing anchor of Kinesio® strip with no tension at start, hold anchor to ensure no tension is added to the base.

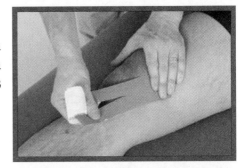

Apply tension to the tape in the direction/opposite direction fascia correction is desired. Moderate to severe tension, (25-75% of available) is applied with minimal inward pressure. The desired effect is to "hold" the myofascial release technique in the desired position.
This can also be accomplished by using the tails to hold the myofascial release as described in mechanical correction.

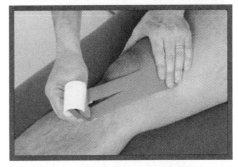

Lay the tails of the tape down with no tension. The tails should be splayed out to dissipate the created tension over as large an area as possible.

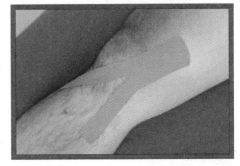

SPACE CORRECTION

The space correction is applied to create more space directly above an area of pain, inflammation, swelling, or edema.   The increased space that is created decreases pressure by lifting the skin directly over the treatment area.

The resulting decreased pressure assists in reducing the amount of irritation on the chemical receptors, thus decreasing pain. An increased level of circulation is also felt to occur in the area, allowing for increased removal of exudate. Stimulation of the mechanoreceptors may also aid in decreasing pain. By increasing sensory stimulation, the gate control theory of pain may be initiated.

Space is created by using the elastic qualities of the Kinesio® Tex Tape to lift fascia and soft tissue over the area of pain or inflammation.   Tape application needs to be performed slowly, and the practitioner should not allow the skin to bunch (can cause a blister) under the Kinesio® Tex Tape or allow the technique to be applied with too much tension (causing irritation to the skin).

The space correction technique may be selected by the practitioner as a primary therapeutic technique following initial evaluation of the patient's condition.   The patient may initially receive the greatest benefit from reduction of inflammation and pain. Following initial reduction in inflammation and pain, the practitioner may select another therapeutic technique such as fascia correction or mechanical correction.

There are four main techniques used with space correction. One, the elastic qualities of the Kinesio® I-Strip can be used to pull the connective tissue toward the desired area by applying the Kinesio® strip with tension out of the middle of the strip with no tension on the ends (modification of ligament and tendon correction). Multiple layers can be used depending upon the size of the area. Two, practitioners can utilize a manual therapy technique to gently gather the skin and fascia and use the Kinesio® Tex Tape to maintain the tissue over the desired area (fascia manual winding technique, see fascia correction technique). Three, practitioners can use fascia correction technique to create and hold tissue over the desired area (see fascia correction technique). Four, practitioners can use the "donut hole" or web cut.

SPACE CORRECTION APPLICATION TECHNIQUES: I-STRIP

Application of Kinesio® "I" strip for space correction: This technique uses the elastic qualities of the Kinesio® Tex Tape to lift the skin and create space. This is accomplished by applying tension to the middle 1/3 section of the Kinesio® strip and laying down both ends with no tension. A single strip or a series of overlapping strips can be applied. With this method, a "pocket" is formed under the tape, decreasing pressure and pain.

Generally an "I" strip is used for this technique. Cut the Kinesio® strip to desired length, generally 6-8 inches. Tear the Kinesio® Tex Tape paper backing in the middle of the strip. Fold back the paper and apply tension to the middle 1/3 of the Kinesio® strip.

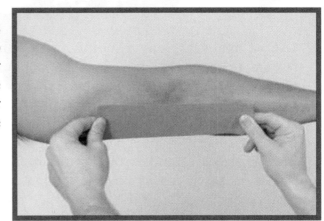

Apply light to moderate tension, (15-50 % of available) to the Kinesio® "I" strip in the middle 1/3 of the strip. Place the center of the Kinesio® strip over the region of the desired space correction. A series of strips can be applied, with the intersection of each strip located over the desired space correction location (area of desired "pocket"). If multiple strips are used, decrease tension applied to each strip to limit accumulation of excess tension.

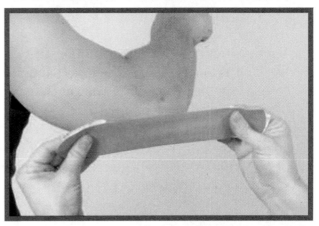

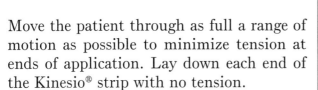

Move the patient through as full a range of motion as possible to minimize tension at ends of application. Lay down each end of the Kinesio® strip with no tension.

Convolutions of the skin should be evident during joint range of motion. If convolutions are not present, the tape was applied with too much tension.

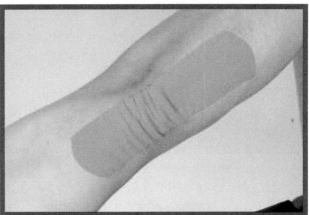

SPACE CORRECTION APPLICATION TECHNIQUES: FASCIA CORRECTIONS USED FOR SPACE CORRECTION

Additional methods of space correction application: These are fascia correction techniques with the desired therapeutic goal of pain and inflammation reduction. The basic facia correction application technique does not change, only the therapeutic goal changes. For complete explanation of each technique refer to Fascia Correction.

Use of manual fascia winding or myofascial release technique: Following the application of a manual therapy technique, position the fascia/skin in the desired position prior to tape application. With this application, the desired therapeutic goal is space correction. Effects on fascia may be a secondary therapeutic result. For review, see fascia correction. The region of space correction should be at the base of the tails.

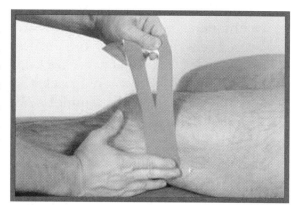

Use of fascia correction technique to reposition fascia: In this technique, the practitioner is going to use the elastic qualities of the Kinesio® Tex Tape to simulate a manual therapy technique. With this application, the desired therapeutic goal is space correction. Effects on fascia may be a secondary therapeutic result. For review, see fascia correction.

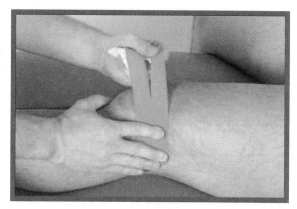

Use of a Kinesio® "I" strip of approximately 6-8 inches with light tension, (15-25% of available, or paper off tension). The tension is added to the middle 1/3 region of the Kinesio® "I" strip. Begin the strip with no tension, and have the patient move the joint or tissue to be treated into a stretched position. As the patient moves into an active motion, lay down the Kinesio® "I" strip with light tension.
If the application is applied correctly, convolutions in the skin will be present.

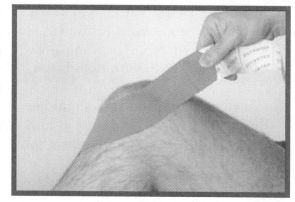

SPACE CORRECTION: HOLE AND WEB TECHNIQUE

This technique uses a hole cut in the center of the Kinesio® "I" strip slightly larger than the area to be treated. The two ends are cut into three tails of approximately 1/3 of the length of the Kinesio® strip. The hole is placed directly over the area in which space is to be created. Light to moderate tension, (15-50 % of available) is applied to the Kinesio® strip prior to placement on the patient while they are in the stretched position. The tails are laid down with no tension to dissipate any force created during tape application.

Hole Technique

Begin by cutting a hole in the center of an approximately 6 inches Kinesio® "I" strip. Be careful to not cut more than 1/2 of the available width of the Kinesio® Tex Tape. This will maximize its ability to adhere to the patient's skin.
Cut approximately 2 inches of each end into two or three strips.

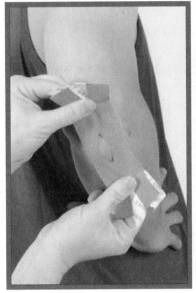
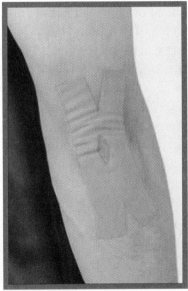

Place the joint into a maximally stretched position as pain and swelling allow. Initially this may be a limited ROM, however as pain and swelling are reduced ROM will improve.
In the center of the Kinesio® strip tear the paper backing and peel back to allow for tension to be applied to the Kinesio® Tex Tape. Apply light to moderate tension, (25-50% of available) to the Kinesio® strip and place the hole directly over the area of desired space. If more than one strip is applied, use light tension.

Lay down the tails on both ends with no tension. Splay the ends to dissipate tension which was created in the area of the donut. Initiate glue activation prior to any patient movement.

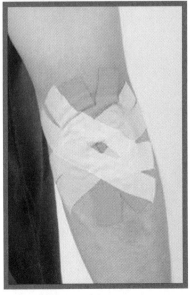

Web Cut

Cut the appropriate length of tape, and fold the tape in half. Cut the Kinesio® strip into 4 - 8 strips, leaving 1 inch at each ends uncut. Begin by placing the joint into a maximally stretched position as pain and swelling allow. Two methods can be used. One: begin by applying one end of the web cut with no tension below the area to be treated. Remove the web strips using paper off tension and apply the second base. Two: tear the paper backing at the center of the fan cut and peel back the paper backing. Apply very light

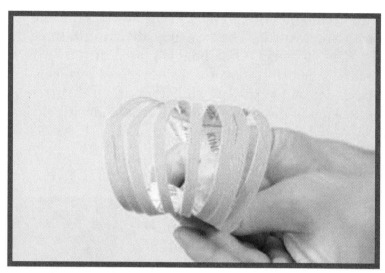

to light tension, (10-25% of available) in the center area of the web cut. As best as you can, separate the web fan strips, so there is approximately 1/4 inch separation. Place the web fan strips over the desired treatment area. Lay down the ends with no tension.

Initiate glue activation prior to any patient movement.

LIGAMENT/TENDON CORRECTION

The ligament/tendon correction is applied to create increased stimulation over the area of a ligament or tendon resulting in increased stimulation to the mechanoreceptors. This stimulus is believed to be perceived as proprioceptive stimulation that is interpreted by the brain as more similar to normal tissue tension.

Kinesio® Tex Tape is applied for ligaments with moderate to severe tension (25-75% of available) with the tape directly over the area of the ligament. Maximum or full tension, (100% of available) may also be used if the practitioner determines it appropriate. The ends of the tails, as always, have no tension at the start or end of the tape application. It can either be applied from origin to insertion or insertion to origin, as determined by the practitioner. Generally, the tape should be applied from insertion to origin; in this manner the tension of the tape will be limiting the allowable movement of the ligament. (It may be desirable to have the patient move the area being taped through a limited or full range of motion if appropriate for function.)

Two methods of application for the ligament/tendon can be used. One: begin by applying the Kinesio® "I" strip with no tension at the beginning; apply desired tension over the length of the ligament; and then lay down the end of the strip with no tension. Second: begin by tearing the paper backing in the middle of the "I" strip. Apply desired tension to the middle 1/3 of the strip, then with tension held in the Kinesio® strip apply the strip over the length of the ligament. End the application by having the patient move the body part through as much range of motion as possible and apply ends of strip with no tension.

Tape application for the tendon is similar, except that less tension, (50% of available) is applied directly over the area of the tendon. In the extreme case, severe (50-75%) tension may be applied. The ends of the tails, as always, have no tension at the start or end of the tape application. Tension can be increased directly over the area of the tendon. When the tape crosses over the muscle belly, the tension should be adjusted for either an origin to insertion (very light tension, 15% of available), or insertion to origin (light to moderate tension, 15-50% of available) application.

LIGAMENT CORRECTION APPLICATION TECHNIQUE

Use of ligament correction technique application to create increased stimulation over the area of a ligament resulting in increased stimulation to the mechanoreceptors: Generally, the base of the corrective strip should be started at the insertion of the ligament. This should ensure the tension being created by the Kinesio® strip has a shortening effect on the skin and joint.

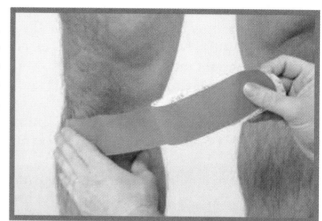

Apply base of tape with no tension. Hold the tape base to ensure that no tension is added. Practitioner may want to practice the placement of the Kinesio® strip prior to base placement to limit error on initial application.

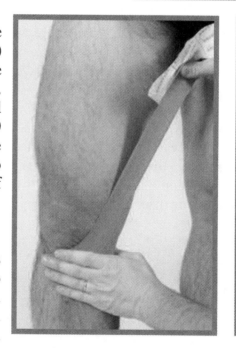
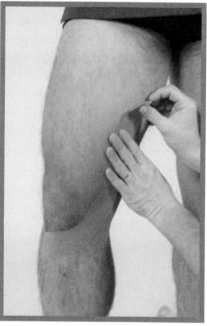

Apply moderate to severe tension, (25-75% of available) along the approximate position of the ligament, with patient in a functional position (e.g. knee 20-30 degrees of flexion). The practitioner may use up to 100% of available tension, if appropriate

Slide the hand that was holding tension at the base up to the end of tension position at approximately the origin of the ligament. Lay down the tail of the tape with no tension. Prior to completion of the Kinesio® strip application, the joint may need to be moved through a full range of motion. Example: for the wrist corrective strip applied in neutral position, tails may be applied during flexion or extension.

TENDON CORRECTION APPLICATION TECHNIQUE

Use of tendon correction technique application to create increased stimulation over the area of a tendon that results in increased stimulation to the mechanoreceptors:
The proper application of the tendon correction technique will have an increased tension, moderate to severe (25-75% of available tension) over the length of the tendon. Tape applied beyond the tendon should be appropriate for an O to I or I to O application.

Apply end of tape with no tension. Hold the tape end to ensure that no tension will be placed on the base of the tape.

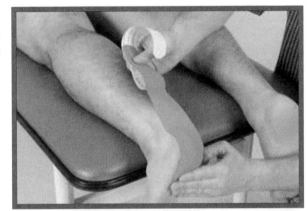

Apply moderate to severe tension, (25-75% of available) along the length of the tendon, with patient in a stretched position. Remember to reduce tension over belly of muscle for either origin to insertion or insertion to origin application.

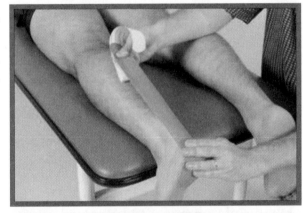

Slide the hand that was holding the base up to the end of tension position. Lay down the base or tails of the tape with appropriate tension for I to O or O to I application. Ligament correction often requires 50-100% tension, and tendon correction 50-75% tension.

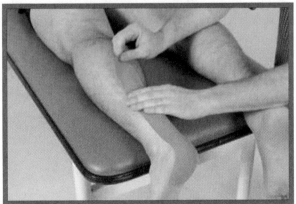

FUNCTIONAL CORRECTION

The functional correction is used when the practitioner desires sensory stimulation to either assist or limit a motion. The Kinesio® Tex Tape is applied to the skin with no tension during active movement. The tension created by the increased stimulation during active movement is believed to provide stimulation to the mechanoreceptors. The perceived stimuli are believed to be interpreted as proprioceptive stimuli, which act as a pre-load during end-of-motion positions.

The Kinesio® Tex Tape is applied by cutting the appropriate length of an "I" strip. Length should be approximately four inches above and below the joint or a length appropriate for the joint chosen. Place the joint or muscle to be taped in the appropriate position. Example: if assisting flexion and resisting extension, place the joint in flexion. Begin tape application at the distal end of selected joint with a minimum of two inches of tape with no tension. Apply appropriate tension (light, moderate, severe or full) then adhere the second base of the tape at the proximal end of the selected joint.

When first using the functional correction, the most difficult part is determining the proper tension during this phase of application. The first time a practitioner applies this technique, do not be surprised if either too much or too little tension is applied. The base should also be a minimum of 2 inches in length with no tension.

With one hand placed on each base, both proximal and distal, have the patient actively move the joint into the opposite range of motion position. Example: if assisting flexion and resisting extension, have the patient now actively move into extension. To finish the tape application, move both hands towards the middle of the joint and apply the remaining tape. Making sure to activate the acrylic glue by rubbing the Kinesio® strip prior to releasing tension on the joint.

Following the functional tape application as described above, the patient will perceive stimuli, which will assist with flexion and resist the end position of extension (in example given). This is accomplished because the mechanoreceptors interpret the stimuli as normal joint position. During extension, the increased tension on the skin will provide a stimulus perceived as reaching the end of normal joint position. This perception is created through increased skin tension which would normally occur at end of motion. Flexion will be assisted as the perception of increased tension in positions of extension causes the repositioning of the joint to normalize perceived skin tension.

FUNCTIONAL CORRECTION APPLICATION TECHNIQUE

Use of functional correction technique to assist or restrict a motion (e.g. flexion or extension). It is believed this is accomplished by changing the perception of joint position through increased tension in the skin. The body will adjust joint position to normalize the increased tension on the skin.

The Kinesio® Tex Tape is applied by cutting the appropriate length of an "I" Strip. Length should be approximately four inches above and below the joint (or a length appropriate for the joint chosen).

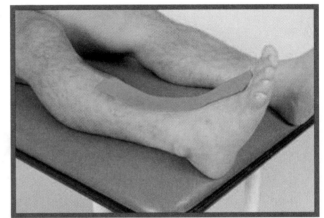

Place the joint or muscle to be taped in the appropriate position. Example: if assisting dorsiflexion and resisting plantar flexion, place the joint in dorsiflexion. Begin tape application at the distal end of selected joint with a minimum of two inches of tape with no tension.

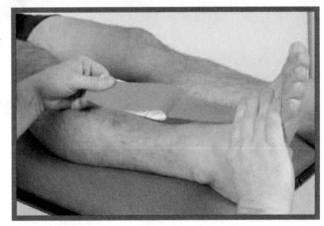

Apply an appropriate degree of tension from light to full and adhere the second base of the tape at the proximal end of the selected joint. Initially it may be difficult to determine the appropriate amount of tension; several applications may be needed prior to establishing proper tension. This base should also be a minimum of two inches of tape with no tension.

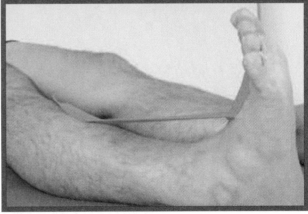

With one hand placed on each base, both proximal and distal, have the patient actively move the joint into the opposite range of motion position. Example: if assisting dorsiflexion and resisting plantar flexion, have the patient now actively move into plantar flexion.

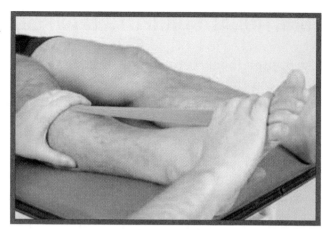

To finish the tape application, move both hands towards the middle of the joint and apply remaining tape. Make sure to activate the acrylic adhesive prior to releasing tension, otherwise the Kinesio® strip will have limited adherence.

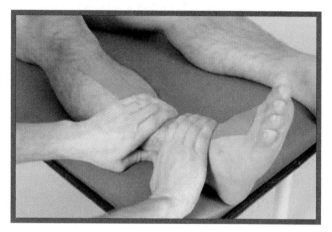

LYMPHATIC CORRECTION

The lymphatic correction is used to assist in the removal of edema by directing fluid towards a less congested lymphatic pathway and lymph node. This is accomplished by the lifting effect and elasticity of Kinesio® Taping. The lifting of superficial skin decreases pressure and opens initial lymphatics, while the tape also creates a massaging action during active motion. The effect of Kinesio® Taping on muscle also improves the efficiency of the deeper lymphatics by allowing maximum contraction and relaxation of a muscle.

The lymphatic system is a one-way system that relies on tissue pressure to assist in movement. During a 24-hour period, between 50 to 100% of plasma proteins leave the blood stream and are taken up by the lymph system. Approximately 2 liters of lymph is processed per day by the body.

Beginning in the superficial dermis at the level of the venous capillaries, the lymphatic system is responsible for the removal of waste products and larger cell proteins that are unable to be transported by the venous system. Interstitial fluid moves into the initial lymph collectors at which time it becomes lymphatic fluid. These initial collectors are extremely small, with flaps or openings that are attached to the skin by small filaments. Movement of skin and pressure changes open and close these vessel openings to allow filling and emptying. Deeper vessels called "lymph angions" lie between muscles and parallel to the venous system. Resembling a "string of pearls", they have one-way valves and utilize a stretch reflex to empty and fill the next angion, creating a type of peristalsis movement of the fluid. Muscle contraction and respiration also assists in propelling lymph throughout the body by creating deep pressure changes.

As lymph moves through the body, it needs to be processed prior to rejoining the venous system and entering the heart. Lymph nodes concentrate and clean the lymph fluid of toxins, dyes, and 'unknown' cells. There are approximately 600 lymph "nodes" in the body, and most are located near organs or major joints of the body. The highest concentration of lymph nodes (160) is found in the neck region. Nodes have an arterial and venous supply that is responsible for increasing the viscosity of the lymph, taking up to 40% of lymphatic fluid content via the capillary circulation. Immune components such as "B" and "T" cells are also located in the lymph nodes, and foreign cells may be destroyed by macrophages or lymphocytes or stored here to be isolated from the body. The concentrated, node-processed lymph then moves into larger deeper lymphatic ducts that are located in the trunk. All ducts join in the upper chest and empty into the left jugular vein prior to returning to the heart.

Edema and inflammation occurs when there is an increase in blood circulation and the lymphatic system is unable to keep up. This may be due to trauma, infection, autoimmune reaction (rheumatoid arthritis), or heat. Inflammation puts pressure on touch receptors. This increased pressure in the superficial layers and lack of skin movement inhibit lymphatic collectors, increasing edema.

* Special thanks to Ruth Coopee OTR-CHT, Vodder MLD-CDT, CKTI for her assistance with this correction technique.

LYMPHATIC CORRECTION APPLICATION TECHNIQUE

Use of lymphatic correction to create space and provide a channel for fluid to move towards lymph node. The Kinesio® strip is applied using a fan cut. Initially it may be easier for the practitioner to use Kinesio® Tex Tape cut into 4 strips. Lymphatic drainage may improve using a fan cut into 5 and even 6 strips.

For lymphatic correction the Kinesio® Tex Tape is cut into approximately 1/4 to 1/2 inch strips, leaving approximately one inch uncut at the base.

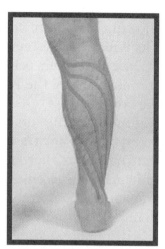

The first Kinesio® Fan Strip applied is a 5-strip cut. Apply the tails of the fan with none to very little tension, (0-15% of available) over area of edema. Place base of fan cut slightly above the lymph node to which lymph drainage is being directed. Have the patient move into a stretch position. In the example shown, the knee is in extension and the ankle in dorsi flexion.

The placement of the lymphatic strips is directed at the appropriate lymphatic duct: photo shows drainage to posterior medial aspect of knee. The second Kinesio® Fan Strip is a 5 cut strip and has been applied in a crisscross pattern.

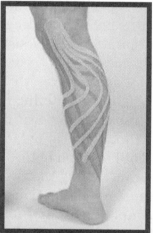

Photo shows drainage to region of Achilles tendon.

Precautions:

KINESIO® TAPING AND DEEP VEIN THROMBOSIS (DVT)
A thrombosis is "the formation, development or existence of a blood clot within the vascular system" (Tabers)
DVT are most often formed in the lower extremities secondary to venous stasis. Post operative, obese and sedentary individuals are in highest danger of developing DVT. They become life threatening if they dislodge move through the heart-resulting in a pulmonary embolism. They may also be found in the upper extremities as well.
Therefore muscle taping is contraindicated if there is any suspicion of DVT.
Superficial Fan Cut taping for edema reduction according to some vascular surgeons is acceptable as it will not affect the tonus of the muscle to dislodge a clot.

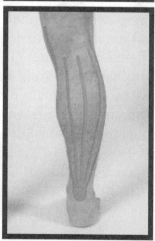

KINESIO® TAPING FOR SCAR TISSUE

Do not apply Kinesio® Tex Tape directly to a scar until it is well healed.

Applying tape too early could cause excessive stress to collagen fiber cross-link formation.

Be extremely cautious with patients with disease processes such as diabetes, venous insufficiency, and peripheral neuropathy.

Scar correction assists in the softening of scar tissue and reducing adhesions and pitting. It helps to make the scar soft, flat, and pliable.

Position patient in maximal muscular and fascia/skin elongation of the scarred area. Lay down an I application to adhere the tape.

Pitting: Position patient in maximal muscular and fascia/skin elongation of the scarred area. Lay down an I tape with 75% stretch. Rub the tape after application to adhere the tape.

Apply cross strip with 75% tension on tape to lift pitted area.

Space Correction:

Increase space by lifting fascia and soft tissue using the elastic quality of the Kinesio® Tex Tape. This will decrease the pressure, reduce irritation on the chemical receptors and decrease pain.

A space correction will assist in decompressing the involved area by utilizing the tape on stretch. The stretched tape will facilitate tissue mobilization over tissue adhesions. Effective over multidirectional adhesions.

Stretch the scar and surrounding tissue

Apply tape stretched in the middle with 30-40% stretch.

Fascia Correction:

Used to gather and hold fascia tissue in the desired position.

Assists in breaking down adhesions and improving tissue movement.

Use inward pressure for a deeper effect.

Fascia connection generally accepted as the most effective in the treatment of scar tissue. Apply tape anchor in the direction of wanted tissue glide, as the natural elastic recoil in the tape will move toward the anchor, directing the fascia. Apply tape with 20-30% stretch. A "Y" application is recommended to dissipate the tension force on the skin. Use more tension when targeting deeper tissue and less tension when targeting superficial tissue.

Begin application in direction of desired tissue movement.

With tissue/muscle on stretch, gather tissue and apply tape with 20-30% stretch.

EVALUATION OF THE CHILD FOR TAPING

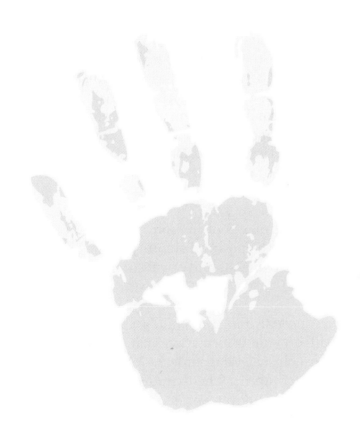

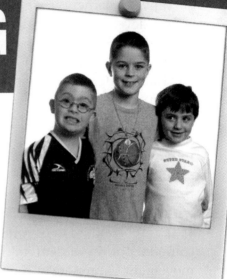

There are a variety of courses and resources available to provide an integrated body of knowledge relevant to treatment techniques for the therapist working with children with disabilities. Presently, there are comprehensive and dynamic approaches to movement education with emphasis on motor learning and motor control, such as the neurodevelopmental treatment approach, proprioceptive neuromuscular facilitation, myofascial release, and constraint induced therapy, to name a few. Effective treatment of children requires a strong knowledge base of infant development and understanding of early motor milestones.[1,2,3] The pediatric therapist must provide a thorough evaluation, management and treatment of the child. The need for carry-over is essential in today's health care. The use of Kinesio® Taping as an adjunctive treatment approach provides input over several days during functional activities, and is key to the success of this intervention.

Clinical observation of the child's movement is critical throughout the assessment. It is important to evaluate the alignment and variety of movement in all positions. The therapist should be knowledgeable of motor development and relate the patterns of movement and posture to the age of the child. Analysis of typical and atypical patterns and postures which interfere with the child's ability to function and move efficiently and effectively is required.

It is important to determine which components of normal movement are present and which components are absent or inefficient. When developing a treatment plan, consider which movement is missing and necessary to perform the functional task. Note what the baby can or cannot do. Emphasis is placed on the quality of movement and what is "normal" or "abnormal" in the pattern of movements of the body. For example, many babies begin to sit independently with their arms free for play by seven or eight months of age. The ability to sit becomes more dynamic as the baby is able to shift weight in all planes of motion. The erector spinae, abdominal, and hip extensor musculature must provide the postural stability to the base of the pelvis for this movement to occur. The baby may lack trunk stability or flexibility and exhibit inefficient patterns to sit erect to free the arm for play.

A basic evaluation of muscle strength, range of motion, and the child's ability to perform functional skills should be performed. This will provide information that is useful for the treatment of the child with neuromuscular and musculoskeletal disorders. Muscle testing is an integral part of the evaluation prior to the child being taped. The therapist must understand motor development, muscle alignment and functional movement to become proficient in the application of Kinesio® Tape. This must include comprehensive knowledge of joint biomechanics, the origin and insertion of muscles, and muscle actions (agonist, antagonist, synergist or fixator).[4,5,6,7] The therapist must observe the muscles in action and recognize the abnormal movements and/or compensatory patterns that occur when muscle weakness exists. The use of Kinesio® Taping can improve biomechanical alignment, assist a weak muscle and provide stability for the child with muscle imbalances.

When one area of the body or muscle is weak, stability of that area is impaired and movement will be altered. Therapists must learn to identify primary concerns and prioritize areas for taping. The pediatric therapist must use clinical observation to evaluate whether or not the Kinesio® Taping technique utilized has helped establish more functional movement. It cannot be over emphasized that a thorough knowledge of motor development in the growing child provides an essential framework for pediatric Kinesio® Taping.

It is hoped that this pediatric Kinesio® Taping book will provide therapists with a useful guide to taping techniques for a wide variety of pediatric conditions. Early identification of patterns of postural malalignment leads to early intervention to correct alignment and muscle imbalances before compensatory patterns are established. Boney modeling forces may also be changed through the achievement of optimal alignment and the facilitation of specific muscle groups through taping, in conjunction with adjunctive treatments. Proper assessment of the infant or child prior to initiating treatment will ultimately maximize the effectiveness of any given treatment approach.

References

1. Alexander R, Boehme R, and Cupps B. 1993. Normal Development of Functional Motor Skills: The First Years of Life. Tucson, Arizona: Therapy Skill Builders.
2. Bly L. 1983. The Components of Normal Movement During the First Year of Life and Abnormal Development. Chicago: Neuro-Developmental Treatment Association.
3. Scherzer AL, and Tscharnuter I. 1982. Early Diagnosis and Therapy in Cerebral Palsy –A primer on infant developmental problems. New York, New York: Marcel Dekker, Inc.
4. Kendall FP, McCreary EK, Provance PG, Rodgers MM, and Romani WA. 2005 Muscles –Testing and Function with Posture and Pain 5th Ed. Baltimore,MD: Lippincott Williams & Wilkins.
5. Calais-Germain B. 1993. Anatomy of Movement. Seattle: Eastland Press.
6. Sieg KW, and Adams SP. 1996. Illustrated Essentials of Musculoskeletal Anatomy. Gainesville, Florida: Megabooks, Inc.
7. Cash M. 1999. Pocket Atlas of the Moving Body. London: Ebury Press.

Suggested Reading

Calais-Germain B. 1993. Anatomy of Movement. Seattle, WA: Eastland Press, Inc.
Cusick B. 1997. Legs & Feet: A Review of Musculoskeletal Assessments. (VHS: 2 hrs) Telluride,CO: Progressive Gaitways, LLC.
Kapandji IA. 1982. The Physiology of the Joints 5th Edition- The Upper Limb, Vol 1. New York: Churchill Livingstone.
Kapandji IA. 1988. The Physiology of the Joints 5th Edition-The Lower Limb, Vol. 2. New York: Churchill Livingstone.
Kapandji IA. 1974. The Physiology of the Joints 2th Edition-The Trunk and the Vertebral Column, Vol. 3. New York: Churchill Livingstone.
Kase K, Wallis J, & Kase T. 2003. Clinical Therapeutic Application of the Kinesio® Taping

Method. Albuquerque, NM. Kinesio® Taping Association.

Muscolino JE. 2005. The Muscular System Manual-The Skeletal Muscles of the Human Body 2nd Ed. St. Louis, MO: Mosby.

Neumann DA. 2002. Kinesiology of the Musculoskeletal System – Foundations for Physical Rehabilitation. St. Louis, MO: Mosby.

Sahrmann SA. 2002. Diagnosis and Treatment of Movement Impairment Syndromes. St. Louis, MO: Mosby.

Soderberg GL. 1986. Kinesiology Application to Pathological Motion. Baltimore, MD: Williams & Wilkins.

KINESIO® TAPING PEDIATRIC SPECIFIC GUIDELINES

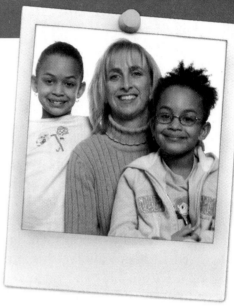

Preparation

The ability to apply Kinesio® Tex tape correctly is important; however a thorough assessment of the child's skin integrity and tape sensitivity is essential to prevent skin reactions. Prior to taping, several factors should be considered. As many children have sensitive skin, a taping sensitivity test prior to application is required. A small piece of tape is applied to the skin, usually on the upper back or abdominal area, as the trunk appears to be more sensitive than the extremities. This test patch is applied to the trunk or potential areas to be taped for four to five days prior to initiation of the taping regimen. If the skin reacts to the test patch applied to the upper back or abdominal areas, this should be taken into consideration when determining future tape application. Reactions may include slight redness, raised skin rashes, itching or, in severe cases, blistering. Caregivers need to be educated in proper test patch removal and signs of skin sensitivity, so that information can be shared with the therapist.

After the child's skin has been tested and it is safe to start taping, prepare the skin areas to be taped. For better adhesion, instruct the caregiver to use mild soap and water to remove oils or lotions from the child's skin in the areas to be taped. Babies and children with sensitive or fragile skin may require a protective skin barrier or commercially available skin prep product. A buffer medium such as Milk of Magnesia can be applied over the skin surface of children with tape sensitivity or fragile skin. Milk of magnesia is a viscous white, mildly alkaline mixture that is used as an antacid and laxative. Although it is not intended for skincare, it has been used in hospitals for this purpose. A light coat of Milk of Magnesia is applied using gauze or a cotton ball and once dried, the excess powder is wiped off. The Kinesio® Tape will not adhere if the coating is too thick. (Some literature suggests that the milk of magnesia can be used as a remedy for clearing up persistent rash, diaper rash, acne and as a facial mask for oily skin.[1,2,3,4]) Clinical judgment should be used on whether the infant or child requires the use of a protective skin barrier. Consult the child's physician, if appropriate, before using. Always consult a physician when using a skin preparation product and taping in a neonatal intensive care unit.

The adhesive backing in the Kinesio® Tex Tape is heat sensitive; and once applied, the tape needs to be rubbed to activate the glue. Before applying the tape, round off the edges of the anchor and tails to prevent the tape from peeling off or getting caught when donning and doffing clothes. If the tape starts to peel off, trim the edges of the tape and allow the rest of the tape to remain on the skin. Do not use a blow dryer as the adhesive is heat sensitive and removal will be more difficult.

The child can take a bath or shower with the tape on. Though some tapes are labeled waterproof and some not, all types can be worn in the bath or shower. Care must be given when drying the child to gently blot the tape with a towel. Children who experience excessive perspiration, live in warm humid climates, or are involved in swim programs may require the use of the waterproof tape.

Precautions

Following tape application, the child's caregiver must be given information on tape removal, signs of skin sensitivity and, if appropriate, application techniques to be done at home. Circumferential taping should be avoided as it may compromise circulation. Warning signs include tingling, pain, paresthesia, or swelling. If these problems occur, removal of the tape is essential. Reddened areas near taped edges may indicate a skin reaction. Itching, pulling at tape or increased irritability may be signs of skin sensitivity. These signs also indicate the tape was applied improperly or with too much tension. Bruising will occur at the edges of tape if applied with excess tension.

Written instructions, including precautions and removal procedures, should be given to the caregivers following tape application (see appendix for taping instruction sheet). The following is a list of concerns to consider when taping:

- A superficial skin reaction may occur in response to adhesive products used on children with sensitive skin. Therefore a skin barrier may be required.
- Wrinkles of the tape on the skin may cause blisters or increased areas of pressure.
- Excessive traction on the anchor may cause bruising or skin breakdown; therefore, the tape should never be pulled taut at either end.
- Perspiration can become trapped between the adhesive and the skin causing a rash which may appear raised and or reddened.
- Skin redness and rash can occur after tape has been worn intermittently for several weeks or months. Constant monitoring of the skin is important. Apply the tape to a different area to prevent skin irritation.
- Use proper removal techniques. The epidermis may remain attached to the adhesive resulting in epidermal damage. Gently pull the skin away from the tape, in the direction of hair growth, during tape removal.
- Skin tears, resulting in blistering, may occur if tape is applied with excess tension.
- An adhesive spray can be used prior to applying the tape for use in sports. When using a spray adherent, it is important to remove the tape immediately after the game. If left on, the chemical irritants from the adhesive spray can become trapped between the adhesive and the skin. A child may have a reaction to the adhesive, exacerbated by the heat generated under the tape.
- Be aware of swelling and edema in the area before and after taping.
- Children with decreased sensation need to be monitored more closely, as they may not be aware of a skin reaction.
- Children with vascular disease or circulatory issues must have skin color and swelling monitored closely.
- Changes in skin pigmentation may occur with taping, though these are usually temporary.
- Never tape over an infected area

Contraindications

- Open wounds
- Fragile skin
- Poor skin integrity
- Abrasions
- Tape allergies

Application

The amount of tension applied to the Kinesio® Tex tape will depend on the specific taping techniques, as described in this book. The stretch placed on the tape will vary according to the amount of tension that is required to assist the muscle, support the joint, ligament, or tendons; or provide a fascial release. In all tape applications, the proximal and distal ends of the tape should have no tension (0-5%), and tension should be placed only in the center of the tape. The anchor is the proximal portion of the tape (generally ½ inch or 1 inch for children) and the tails are the distal portion of the tape. The tails will generally rebound or shrink back toward the anchor. An example of this is to apply the Kinesio® Tex tape to treat a painful or cramped muscle. The tape is applied from insertion to origin with the muscle in the elongated position. The tape is initially applied at the anchor with no tension (0-5%), and then applied with paper off, light tension which is 10%-15%, and end with ½ inch or 1 inch with no tension (0-5%).

The tape is at a 10% stretch when removed directly from the paper and onto a muscle, and this is called paper-off or light tension. Tape applications in this book, will include indicated tension to be placed on the tape, as well as position of the body part to be taped. Tension of the tape will go from no tension to maximal, which is used often for supporting ligaments and over areas of pain.

The guidelines below describe the amount of tension or stretch used when applying the Kinesio® Tex tape on children. The therapist must recognize that the tension applied on the tape will vary according to the ability of the infant or child to tolerate the input from the tape. The comfort level and reaction to the tape application may indicate how much stretch the child will be able to handle and may require adjustments. Specific tension mentioned in techniques may also vary, based on clinical findings.

No tension	0-5%
Minimal (Paper-off)	10-15%
Minimal to moderate	15-25%
Moderate	25-50%
Moderate to Maximum	50-75%
Maximum (Full)	75-100%

- Origin to insertion: use paper-off (minimal) tension of 10%-15%, though tension may be effectively increased by shortening the muscle facilitated.
- Insertion to origin: use paper-off (minimal) tension of 10-15%.

Corrective Applications

- **Mechanical Correction**: uses paper-off (light) to moderate tension (10%-25%). The mechanical correction technique is used to assist with postural alignment. When taping adults, maximal stretch may be used to provide stimulus perceived by the mechanoreceptors. This technique is used to assist in the positioning of muscle, fascia, tissue or joint position. For children the mechanical correction technique is applied with light to moderate tension (10%-25%). The child is initially positioned in better biomechanical alignment, and taped in this corrected position. Children appear to tolerate wearing this tape, using less tension than the adult.
- **Fascia Correction**: uses paper-off (light) to moderate tension (10%-25%).
- **Space Correction**: uses moderate to maximal tension (50%-75%), maximal tension (75%-100%).
- **Ligament/ Tendon Correction**: uses moderate to maximal tension (50%-75%), maximal tension (75%-100%).
- **Functional Correction**: moderate (25%-50%), moderate to maximal (50%-75%). Full or maximal stretch (100%) is rarely used for this technique in children, as they may not tolerate the full stretch. Increased support is provided by placing the muscle facilitated in a shortened position.

Application Specifics

After tape application, always rub tape to adhere the glue.

Never apply tension at the anchor or end of the tape.

The amount of tension applied to the tape and the position of the body segment to be taped, are determined by the results desired. For example:
- muscle facilitation
- more optimal muscle alignment
- fascial release
- improvement of joint position
- stabilization of a joint
- improvement of function

Increased force of the tape can be achieved in four ways
- taping a muscle/ joint in a shortened position
- increased tension on the tape
- wider tape
- tape over tape

If you are able to achieve desired results with minimal to moderate assist of your hands, Kinesio® Tape application may be used. If moderate to maximal force is required, Kinesio® Tex tape will not be as effective, or may cause skin breakdown.

Removal

Kinesio® Tex tape will begin to lose its elasticity after three to four days, though it may be worn for up to six days. Instruct the caregiver to remove the tape the night before new tape is reapplied to let the skin breathe before applying more tape. In some cases, such as in a ligament strain or tear, the tape needs to be removed only a short time before reapplication and the skin should be more closely monitored. If skin sensitivity is present, the wearing schedule may be adjusted accordingly. For example, the tape may be worn for two days on and one day off before reapplying.

For ease of removal, apply baby oil, vegetable oil, or lotion on the tape for fifteen minutes before taking off the tape. Removal in the bath or shower is effective. While in the shower or bath, slowly take off the tape by carefully pulling the skin away from the tape. Roll the tape off close to the skin, being careful not to lift the skin. Remove the tape along the direction of the hair line. Never rip off the tape, as this will cause tearing of the skin and abrasions.
After tape removal, clean the skin with warm, soapy water. Lotion may be applied to skin, though not immediately before reapplication of tape.

References

1. Mussehi, J (2003). Experts: Makeup and Skincare. Retrieved from http://experts.about.com/q/1434/3262001.htm
2. Magnesia Mud Mask. (n.d.). Bottle of rain: a site on home, garden, health, cooking, collecting and everything else. Retrieved from http://bottleofrain.blar.org/bottleofrain.pl?user_record=%2255%22
3. Phillips Milk of Magnesia. (2004). Retrieve November 12, 2004, from http://kdkaradio.com/content/content.cgi?database=Logue%20Content.db&command=vi
4. Brattain, E. (n.d.). Nursery Tips Nappy/Diaper Rash. Retrieved from http://www.hinsandthings.co.uk/nursery/tips.htm

HEAD AND NECK

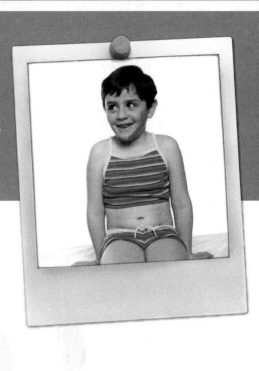

Cervical Alignment

This technique is used to facilitate capital flexion and improved alignment of the head on the trunk.

Trunk alignment may need to be addressed prior to this application. If the thoracic spine is flexed, the cervical spine may be positioned in increased extension, allowing the child to look forward.

This technique is also useful to improve neck stability and to support hypermobility at lower cervical levels. This may also decrease pain or strain in the cervical area.

A 2 inch "Y" tape, a 2 inch "I" tape

- Observe position of neck and trunk from all directions
- Measure the tape length from the occiput to the T2 spinous process

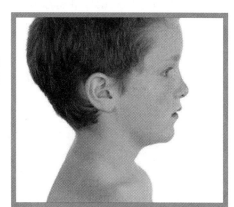

- Cue the patient to flex the neck at each vertebral level, to obtain a chin tuck position, and elongating the capital extensors
- Use tactile cues along each vertebral segment, accompanied by verbal cues to "flex from here"
- Head should stay in "chin tuck" position during taping

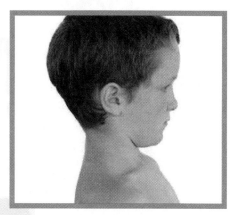

- The first piece of tape is applied insertion to origin, in a lengthened position

- Anchor the base of the "Y" at the occiput
- If the hairline is low, patient may need to be shaved to provide optimal support

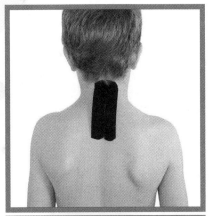

- Apply the tape past the level of restriction, with paper-off tension
- Apply one tail at a time, while continuing to cue the patient to maintain the chin tuck position
- Tails should extend past the second thoracic vertebra

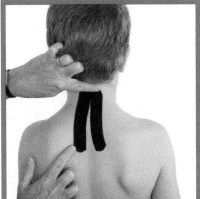

Mechanical Correction tape

- Head should stay in "chin tuck" position during taping
- Tear the tape backing and fold back the edges
- The tape is applied, with full tension on the center of the tape, at level of hypermobile segment
- No tension is applied at the end of the tape

Tension on this correction tape is dependent on evaluation and hypermobility in the cervical spine

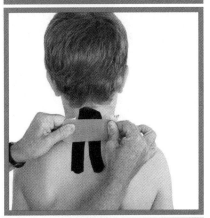

- The correction piece is applied to increase cervical stability
- Correction piece must not be long enough that it limits neck rotation
- Multiple correction tapes may be applied, beginning with superior and overlapping subsequent inferior pieces of tape by ½ inch
- Completed taping for cervical alignment

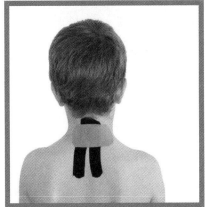

Sternocleidomastoid

Kinesio® Tex tape can be used to assist in facilitating overlengthened muscles and promoting optimal alignment in infants and children with torticollis. Tape is applied to the overlengthened sternocleidomastoid (SCM) muscle. Tape can be applied origin to insertion, or insertion to origin. Tape application to the overlengthened SCM from mastoid to clavicle (insertion to origin) is often effective to facilitate the muscle. The rationale for the effectiveness of taping insertion to origin can include the sensory input from the tape, facilitating the SCM. Input from the visual system also orients to midline and the head may be considered a functional origin in aligning posture to upright and providing midline orientation. Limitation in the SCM in children with torticollis may also increase neck extension, due to weak deep neck flexors.

Soft tissue extensibility in the shortened SCM, scalenes, splenius capitus, upper trapezius, and fascial system needs to be addressed prior to taping the overlengthened muscles. In the treatment of torticollis, Kinesio® Tex tape may also be applied to the upper trapezius, from insertion to origin in the lengthened position (acromion to mastoid and horizontally to the spinous process of the scapula. Kinesio® Tex tape can also be applied to facilitate the lower and middle trapezius.)

Sternocleidomastoid

Origin: sternum (one head) and medial third of the clavicle
Insertion: mastoid
Action: neck lateral flexion toward the same side, rotation toward the opposite side

Taping to facilitate overlengthened SCM and provide sensory input.

A 1 inch "Y" tape (older child), a ½ inch "I" or "Y" tape (infant)

If torticollis is present, taping of OVERLENGTHENED SCM is indicated

- To identify the SCM, neck should be rotated to the opposite side and laterally flexed toward the same side
- Measure tape length from mastoid process to the sternoclavicular joint, on overlengthened side

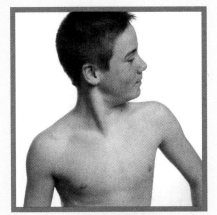

- Anchor tape at the SCM origin (sternoclavicular joint and medial third of the clavicle)
- Apply medial and lateral tails toward the mastoid, with paper-off tension
- On an infant, SCM may be so small that ½ inch "I" strip of tape may be used
- This technique works well for infants under six months and may be done using an "I" tape.

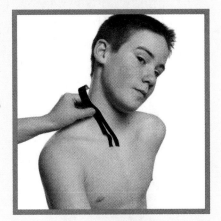

- Apply tape with paper-off tension to mastoid process
- No tension is applied at the end of the tape

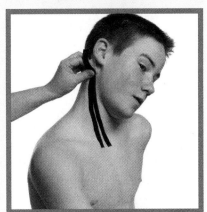

- Completed taping for overlengthened sternocleidomastoid
- Evaluate head position and movement in all positions after taping

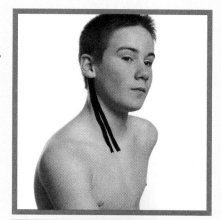

Alternate taping:
(insertion to origin)

- Anchor tape at mastoid process
- Maintain SCM in elongated position to apply tape.
- If tape is not effective to assist in midline head position and SCM contraction, tape may be applied with SCM in less lengthened position the next session
- Gradual improvement may be observed weekly

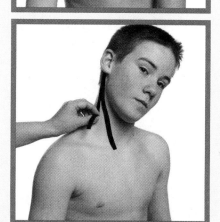

- Apply the medial tail toward the sternoclavicular joint, with paper-off tension
- No tension is applied at the end of the tape

- Apply lateral tail towards the medial third of the clavicle, with paper-off tension
- No tension is applied at the end of the tape
- May be used for infants and children over six months of age, as visual system orients head to neutral and may act as functional origin or point of stability. Assess if this technique is more effective than taping origin to insertion.

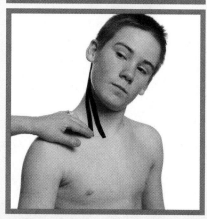

Anterior Scalene Taping

Kinesio® Tex tape may also be applied to the overlengthened scalene muscles if an asymmetric head tilt is evident, as in torticollis. Kinesio® Tex tape can be applied from origin to insertion. There are three defined scalene muscles, anterior, middle, and posterior. In infants with torticollis, it may be best to focus on taping the overlengthened anterior and/or middle scalene, as deep neck flexors are not fully developed and tape on the posterior cervical area may facilitate unwanted neck extension.

This taping is often done in conjunction with taping of the over-lengthened SCM for infants with torticollis. The brachial plexus and the subclavian artery pass between the anterior and middle scalene.

Anterior Scalene

Origin: anterior tuberosities of the transverse processes of the third through sixth cervical vertebrae
Insertion: medial 2/3rds of the first rib
Action: The scalenus group act unilaterally as lateral flexors of the neck and bilaterally as flexors of the cervical spine. At the same time, these muscles greatly influence the respiratory muscles

"I" tape 1 inch width, or smaller for infant

- This taping technique is often used in conjunction with SCM taping for the infant and child with torticollis
- Tape is applied to the overlengthened side
- Measure tape length from transverse processes of cervical spine to just below the clavicle
- Position the neck in slight elongated position, or neutral
- Position of head will help determine the amount of input from the tape
- For more input, place head in more neutral and less elongated position

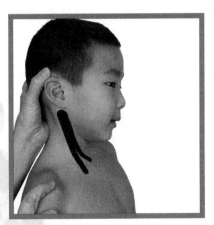

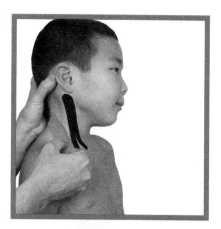

- Anchor the tape on the transverse processes of the cervical vertebrae

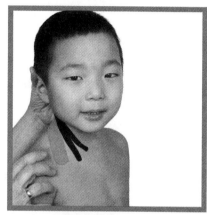

- Apply tape with paper-off tension in a diagonal toward the middle of the clavicle

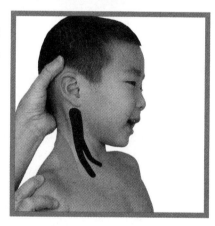

- Completed taping to facilitate and provide input to overlengthened anterior and middle scalene, in conjunction with SCM taping

Lip Closure

Head and Neck

Orbicularis Oris

Origin: alveolar border of maxilla lateral to midline of mandible
Insertion: circumferentially around mouth, blending with other muscles
Action: closes the lips / protrudes the lips

Facilitation of Lip Closure:

The orbicularis oris is the major muscle responsible for lip closure. In children with neuromuscular involvement, this is generally a weakened muscle, due to overstretch from poor closure, head and neck position and poor alignment, and muscle imbalances.

Taping with this method has been shown to improve "pursing of lips" and mouth closure. Children do tire and initial tape is worn for a maximum of 45 minutes, with time gradually increased.

The mechanism of impact may be primarily sensory, due to input directly over the orbicularis oris or may involve facilitation of the orbicularis oris muscle itself.

Two ½ to ¾ inch "I" tapes

- Measure tape length needed to fit around the mouth when it is fully opened
- Instruct child to keep mouth open
- Tear tape backing at center of first piece, and fold back edges
- Anchor tape at the center of mouth, above upper lip

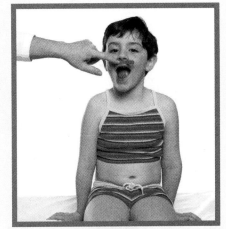

- While the mouth is open, lay down the tape with paper-off tension
- Tape should end at corners of upper lip
- Do not place tape on lips, but just outside of lips, outlining mouth

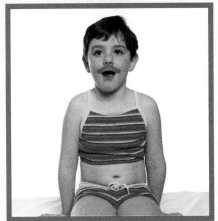

- Take second piece of tape and anchor at center of lower lip
- Tear tape backing at center of second piece of tape, and fold back edges
- Anchor tape at the center of mouth, below lower lip
- With mouth open, lay down tape with paper-off tension

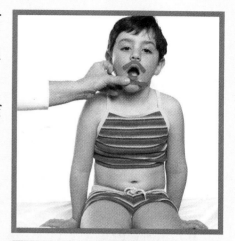

- Tape should surround the mouth, following the orbicularis oris muscle
- The tape ends should overlap slightly
- No tension at the end of the tape
- Completed taping for lip closure

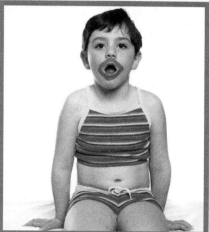

Jaw Stability

Children with neuromuscular involvement often have decreased jaw stability and difficulty grading movement of the jaw for chewing. Kinesio® Tape can be applied to assist in improving jaw control and stability for speech and eating.

This technique is usually done bilaterally, for symmetrical jaw stabilization.

A 1.5 to 2 inch "Y" cut, with superior tail shorter than inferior tail

- Measure tape length from TMJ to mandible
- To cut both pieces simultaneously, place them back-to-back, and cut "Y" with one tail shorter than the other
- Anchor the tape at the TMJ joint

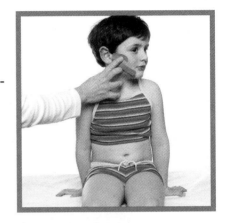

- Apply the superior tail with paper-off tension, diagonally along upper jaw and cheek

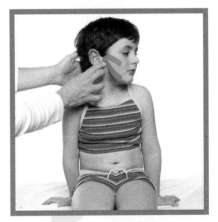

- Instruct the child to open mouth, but observe to be sure jaw does not sublux or retract
- Apply the inferior tail with paper-off tension to the mandible
- The inferior tail can be longer, to provide additional sensory input to the jaw
- No tension is applied at the end of the tape

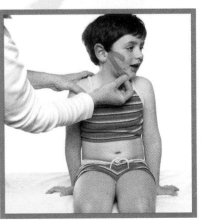

- Repeat taping to opposite side, applying the same tension to tape

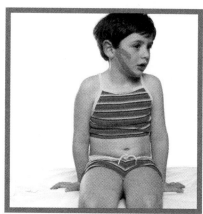

- Completed taping for jaw stability

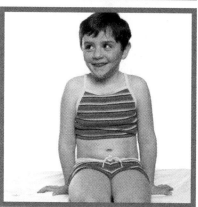

Tempromandibular Joint Stabilization

The temporomandibular joint (TMJ) is the articulation between the condyle of the mandible and the squamous portion of the temporal bone.
The condyle is elliptically shaped with its long axis oriented mediolaterally.
Prior to taping this joint with Kinesio® Tex tape, a thorough evaluation of TMJ movement is essential; as potential to cause increased pain is possible. TMJ involvement may cause headaches, difficulty chewing bruxism (teeth grinding), and pain.

Two ½ to ¼ inch "I" tapes, about 1 to 2 inches long

- Locate TMJ joints and palpate movement
- Identify which, if any, is hypermobile
- The painful joint may be hypermobile, hypomobile, or the pain may be for a variety of other reasons
- Determine if one or both TMJ are to be taped
- Tear tape backing in the center and fold back edges

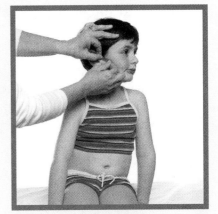

- Tear backing down the center and fold back the edges
- Pull full tension from center of the tape and place diagonally over TMJ joint
- Place a second piece of tape diagonally over first, to form an "X" over the joint
- This technique may be done bilaterally to improve jaw stability
- The "X" may be extended forward toward mouth

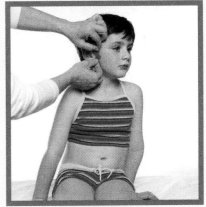

- Completed taping of the tempromandibular joint

Taping a hypermobile joint should follow only after a complete assessment, with instructions to remove tape with any concerns or increase in symptoms

After taping of the TMJ, the following have been observed:
- Decreased drooling
- Improved jaw stability
- Decreased bruxism is some cases
- Improved symmetry of jaw movements.

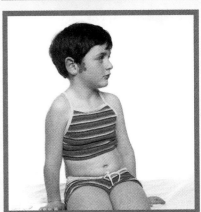

Facial Weakness

Facial weakness, when only part of the face is affected, can occur by trauma to the 7th cranial nerve induced by tumor, surgery, stroke or traumatic brain injury. The degree of facial weakness may vary between individuals due to the location and extent of the damage. The physical symptoms may include an overall droopy appearance or partial facial weakness, asymmetrical smile, facial muscle weakness, difficulty with speaking, eating or drinking. Facial asymmetries may also be seen in children with torticollis or craniofacial anomalies. Kinesio® Taping can minimize the asymmetrical facial appearance and improve the ability to draw the corner of the mouth up to smile, or for lip closure to avoid spillage during eating and drinking.

A 1 inch or ½ inch "Y" tape

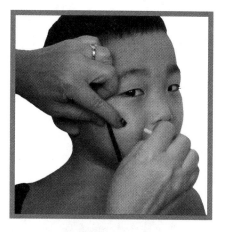

- Measure from the upper cheekbone (zygomatic arch) to just proximal to the upper lip
- Anchor the tape at the upper cheekbone (zygomatic bone)
- This tape follows the zygomaticus minor and major muscles

- Apply minimal tension to the superior tail, applying the tape toward the lateral side of the upper lip

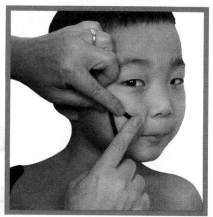

- Apply   minimal   tension   to   the   inferior   tail   to   the   corner

of the lower lip
- No tension is applied at the ends of the tails

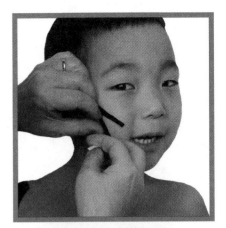

- Completed taping for facial weakness

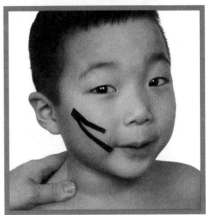

UPPER EXTREMITY

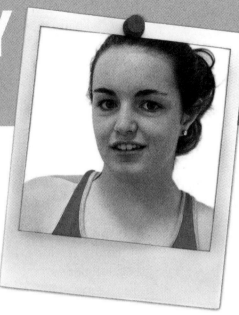

Rhomboids

Origin: C6-7 rhomboid minor, T1-4 spinous processes rhomboid major
Insertion: Medial border of the scapula
Action: Elevates, adducts, and downwardly rotates the scapula

Taping the rhomboids will assist with stabilizing the scapula for children practicing transfer skills from the wheelchair to the mat. The strength of humeral extension and adduction will be supported by the rhomboid tape. The proprioceptive input of the tape will assist with muscle reeducation for children with poor motor control from CVA hemiplegia, traumatic brain injury, and spinal cord injury. Also taping both rhomboids can improve biomechanical alignment of the head on the trunk.

A 1.5 or 2 inch "X" tape

- One way to test or find the rhomboids is to adduct and internally rotate the arm with child's hand over the posteior pelvis
- Then apply counter-pressure as the child attempts to lift the arm away from her body
- Measure the tape length from the spinous processes of C7 to the medial border of the scapula, with the arm in horizontal adduction, in front of the body

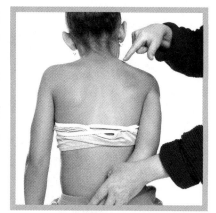

- Tear the paper backing in the center of tape by pulling on both ends to expose the center, and then fold back the edges
- Lay down the center of the tape on a diagonal between the spinous processes and the medial border of the scapula

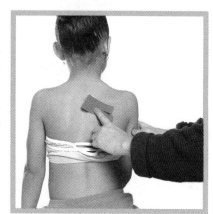

- Position arm in internal rotation and horizontal adduction, toward the opposite leg, with shoulder depressed and protracted
- Apply the tails on an angle, following the rhomboid muscles diagonally, with medial portion of tails higher
- Apply minimal to moderate tension to the tails
- No tension is applied at the end of the tape

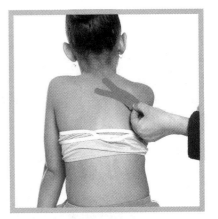

- Completed taping to facilitate the rhomboids

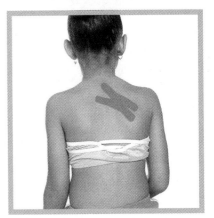

Upper Extremity

Upper Trapezius

Origin: Occiput, nuchal ligament, and C7
Insertion: Lateral 1/3 of the clavicle and acromion
Action: Upper fibers elevates and upward rotates the scapula, elevates the clavicle

The upper trapezius is a commonly overworked muscle, with resulting tightness and shortness of the muscle. Many children with upper trapezius tightness exhibit a forward head and kyphosis of the spine. This may cause symptoms of pain, spasm, muscle stiffness, and headaches. Children often compensate using the upper trapezius to assist with overhead reach. The upper trapezius is short and tight which further causes a muscle imbalance of the force couple of upward rotation of the scapula. The tight upper trapezius can be taped from insertion to origin to relax and lengthen the overworked muscle.

This technique is to elongate the upper trapezius.

A 1.5 or 2 inch "Y" tape

- Measure the tape length from the acromion to the mastoid process, behind the ear lobe
- Anchor the tape at the acromion process

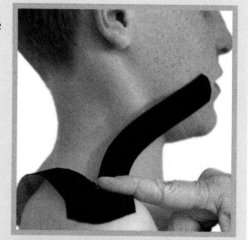

- Side bend the neck toward the opposite side, with slight rotation toward the same side
- Apply the tape with paper-off tension along the upper trapezius, toward the mastoid process

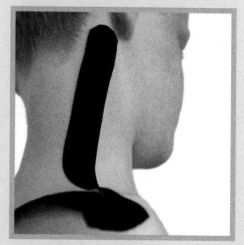

- Position the head back in midline
- With the elbow and shoulder flexed, bring arm to horizontal adduction toward opposite shoulder
- Apply the inferior tail with paper-off tension horizontally toward the spine
- Tape outlines the fascial area of the upper trapezius

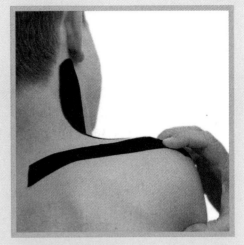

- Completed taping for elongation of the upper trapezius

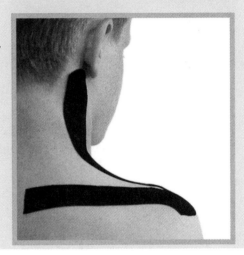

Upper Trapezius Assist

A 1.5 or 2 inch "I" tape

- Measure the tape length from the acromion to the mastoid process, behind ear lobe
- Anchor the tape at the mastoid process

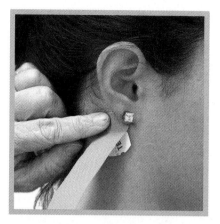

- Neck may be positioned in midline, or with upper trapezius elongated, depending on the amount of assist indicated
- Apply the tape with paper-off tension along the upper trapezius, toward the acromion

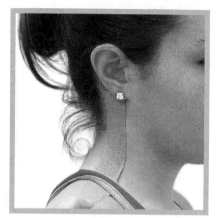

- Completed taping for facilitation of the upper trapezius

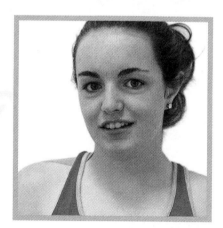

Scapular Stabilization: Middle Trapezius and Lower Trapezius

Middle Trapezius

Origin: T1-T5
Insertion: Acromion and scapular spine
Action: Adduction of the scapula with stabilization of the upper and lower trapezius

Lower Trapezius

Origin: T6-T12
Insertion: Spine of scapula
Action: Depresses the scapula, rotation of the scapula by the upper and lower trapezius with stabilization of the middle trapezius.

If the upper trapezius is shortened and overworked, it places the middle and lower trapezius in the over lengthened and weakened position. The middle and lower trapezius reinforce thoracic spine extension.

Assess the scapular position and alignment on the rib cage. Prior to taping mobilize the scapula to position on the thorax. Combine techniques to perform soft tissue release, for example Myofascial Release (MFR) prior to taping. Lengthen upper trapezius and apply tape to facilitate the middle and lower trapezius to bring the scapula down and in. The scapula is positioned on the thorax between T2- T7-8. The scapula should lie flat against the thorax and in upward rotation.

Two 1.5 or 2 inch "I" tapes

Lower Trapezius:

- Position the child with the trunk in extension and the scapula in alignment chest expanded
- Ask child to "sit up" and bring shoulders "down and back"
- Anchor the tape at T12

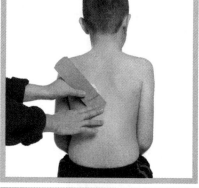

- Maintain the scapula in alignment while applying the tape with paper-off tension
- Apply the tape toward the acromion
- No tension is applied at the end of the tape

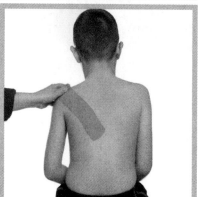

Middle Trapezius:

- Continue to maintain trunk and scapula in alignment
- Anchor the tape at the T2-T3 spinous processes, over the middle trapezius
- Apply the tape with paper-off tension, maintaining scapula optimal alignment
- No tension is applied at the end of the tape

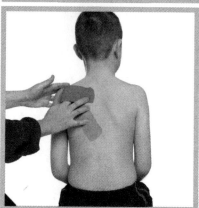

- Completed taping for scapular stabilization

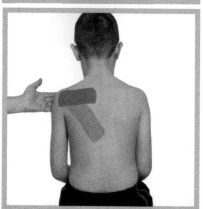

Alternate Lower Trapezius

The "Y" taping technique provides a dynamic stability of the scapula.
Leave 1/3 the lower portion or base of the "Y" and cut tails 2/3 of the length

A 1.5 inch or 2 inch "Y" tape

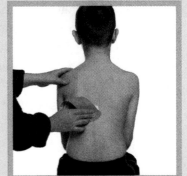

- Measure the tape length from T12 to the acromion
- Identify the scapular borders
- Cue the patient to maintain upright posture with shoulders "down and back"
- Anchor the tape at T12, extending the tape diagonally upward, with no tension on the anchor

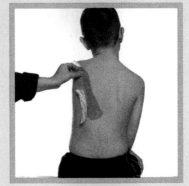

- Apply medial tail with the arm at the side and paper-off tension on the tail as it is applied toward the middle trapezius

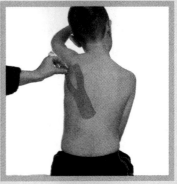

- Abduct and flex the arm, as the lateral tail is applied with paper-off tension to the posterior deltoid, to cue patient to use external rotation as the arm moves into abduction

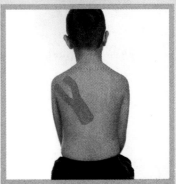

- Completed taping to facilitate the lower trapezius

Subluxed Shoulder

Children with brachial plexus injury, traumatic brain injury, CVA hemiplegia or other conditions may present with varying degrees of muscle imbalance as well as subluxation of the glenohumeral joint. Shoulder subluxation occurs when the muscles of the shoulder girdle are weak or flaccid. An inferior subluxation occurs when the humeral head is located below the inferior lip of the glenoid fossa. The scapula is generally positioned in downward rotation which pulls the humeral head down. An anterior subluxation occurs when the humeral head is positioned in front of the glenoid fossa. The humerus is positioned in internal rotation and forward, the distal end of the humerus moves into hyperextension. Evaluate the position of the scapula and humerus prior to Kinesio® Taping.

Two 1.5, 2 or 3 inch "I" tapes

- Position the humerus in the scapular plane at 45° abduction
- Support the humerus at the elbow with slight compression into the glenoid fossa (Do not jam into position; check the alignment of the scapula)
- Anchor the tape just proximal to elbow crease

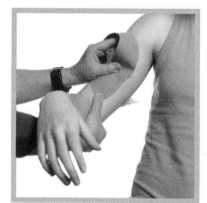

- Apply the tape with moderate tension toward the acromion
- Continue over the acromion with the humeral head positioned

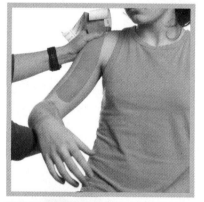

- Apply the tape downward, toward the scapula, to provide support

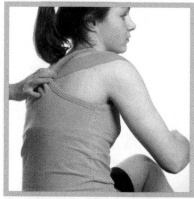

Inferior subluxation: Space correction
- A 2 inch or 1.5 inch I tape
- Measure from coracoid process to spine of scapula
- Continue to provide support at the elbow, to maintain alignment of the humerus
- Tear the tape backing in the center and apply compression in toward the glenoid fossa, with moderate to maximal tension below the humeral head
- No tension is applied on the anchors
- <u>Alternative:</u> tear tape in middle and apply compression below the humeral head with a slight upward "U" curve to assist with holding the humeral head in position (No tension is applied on the anchors)

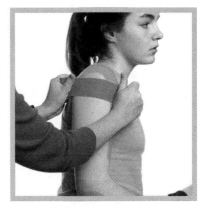

Anterior subluxation : Space correction
A 2 inch or 1.5 inch I tape

- Position the head of the humerus and shoulder girdle in alignment
- Put the arm in slight external rotation
- Anchor tape medial to coracoid process

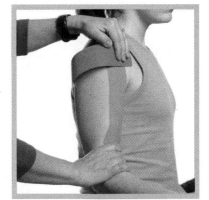

- Apply the tape around the humeral head, with moderate tension
- Apply a force into external rotation, until reaching spine of the scapula with the Kinesio® Tape

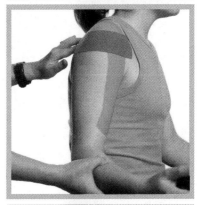

- Completed taping for the subluxed shoulder

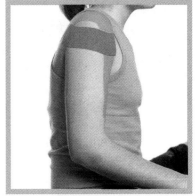

Acromioclavicular Joint Strain

The acromioclavicular (AC) joint is responsible for maintaining the articulation between the clavicle and the scapula during upward rotation of the scapula and elevation of the upper extremity. As the clavicle elevates the coracoclavicular ligaments become taut and rotates the distal end of the clavicle which allows for an additional 30° of scapular rotation. Injury to the AC joint can cause great discomfort when raising the arm into shoulder flexion or abduction greater than 90°. Active overhead movement can be extremely painful with an acromioclavicular joint sprain, complete or partial tearing of the acromioclavicular and coracoclavicular ligaments, or with a possible fracture.

A 2 inch or 1.5 inch "I" tape

- Tape is applied over the area of pain
- Tear the tape backing in the center and fold back edges
- Apply tape with full tension over the center of the acromion

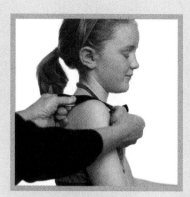

- Lay the anchors of the tape down with no stretch
- Apply anteriorly over the coracoid process and posteriorly near the spine of the scapula

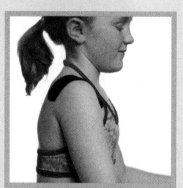

- Lay a second piece of tape down, slightly overlapping the first tape medially
- Apply with full tension from the center of the tape and no tension at the ends, as with the previous piece
- Completed taping

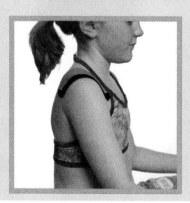

Forward Shoulder

An assessment of the postural muscles of the trunk including the pelvis is important for providing a stable base of support. The stability of the trunk alignment will affect the scapula and clavicle, which has direct muscular and biomechanical effects of the movements of the upper extremity. A forward shoulder girdle may be accompanied by a winged scapula or abducted scapula. The pectoralis minor and clavicular and sternal heads of the pectoralis major muscles may also be tight and shortened.

The Kinesio® Tape is used to assist in positioning the shoulder in better alignment for functional support without losing active range of motion or inhibiting circulation. This may be accomplished in two ways. One is with proper positioning of the area and with added tension during application of the Kinesio® Tape. Another is by correcting the misalignment by using the elastic properties of the Kinesio® Tape to pull the misalignment towards correction.

A 1.5 or 2 inch "Y" tape

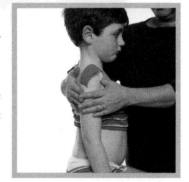

- Prior to tape application, evaluate position of the humerus
- Provide myofascial release, joint mobilization or other treatment technique to relax and position the shoulder girdle
- Position shoulder girdle in alignment prior to application
- Clinically assess where to apply the tails i.e. anchor at the coracoid process with the tails over the shoulder or with the tails more laterally to open up the chest

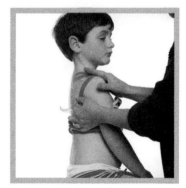

- Measure from the coracoid process to the inferior angle of the scapula or toward the 5th or 6th rib
- Apply the anchor at the coracoid process with no tension

- Angle the tape in the direction for the correction to occur
- Lay down tails of "Y" tape to dissipate force
- Use paper-off tension on the tape and place downward pressure into the skin while applying tape
- No tension is applied at the end of the tape

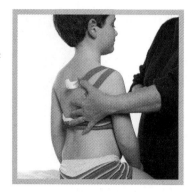

- Maintain postural alignment while applying the other tail
- Use paper-off tension and place downward pressure into the skin
- No tension is applied at the end of the tape
- Completed taping of forward shoulder- postural correction technique

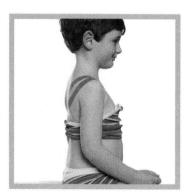

Pectoralis Major

Origin: Clavicle, sternum, 1st to 6th rib
Insert: Greater tubercle of humerus
Action: Adducts and medially rotates the humerus

The pectoralis major attaches directly on the humerus and is a powerful internal rotator of the humerus. This muscle may also contribute to excessive anterior glide of the humeral head. Tightness or increased tone in the pectoralis muscle can restrict elevation of the humerus, a common problem with children with CNS dysfunction. Taping to elongate the pectoralis major muscle may improve upper extremity alignment and promote a more optimal position of the upper extremity. Assess the position of the upper extremity, including position of the anticubital crease, olecranon and thumb, in relation to the body.

Goal: to elongate the pectoralis major muscle

A 1.5 or 2 inch "Y" tape

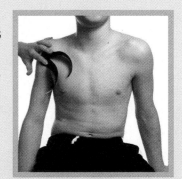

- Measure tape length from the greater tubercle of humerus to 4th rib
- Adhere the tape anchor to the greater tubercle of humerus, located on the proximal humerus with the arm by the side

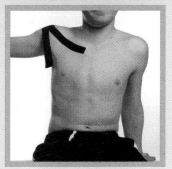

- Position the arm in abduction, external rotation and horizontal extension (elongating the pectoralis major)
- Apply the superior tail with paper-off tension below the clavicle, toward the sternum
- No tension is applied at the end of the tape

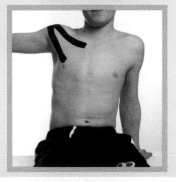

- Apply the inferior tail with paper-off tension along the 4th or 5th rib toward the sternum or toward the nipple
- No tension is applied at the end of the tape
- Completed taping for pectoralis major elongation

Pectoralis Minor

Origin: 3rd to 5th ribs
Insert: Coracoid process of scapula
Action: Tilts the scapula anteriorly, protracts and abducts the scapula

The pectoralis minor lifts the inferior border of the scapula. Tightness of this muscle can contribute to thoracic outlet syndrome by compressing the brachial plexus and axillary artery which runs beneath the muscle. Providing length to the tight muscle through taping can also be counterbalanced by stengthening the antagonist, i.e. the over lengthened lower trapezius.

A 2 inch or 1 ½ inch "Y" tape

- Measure the tape length from the coracoid process to the 4th rib
- Apply the anchor to the coracoid process, with the arm by the side

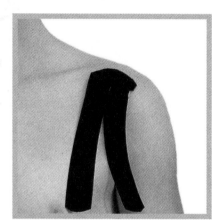

- Position the arm overhead in humeral abduction and external rotation (fully elongate the pectoralis minor)
- Apply the medial tail with paper-off tension, in a downward diagonal direction toward the 3rd or 4th rib
- Apply the lateral tail with paper-off tension in a downward diagonal direction, toward the 5th rib or toward the nipple

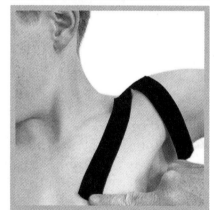

- Completed taping for pectoralis minor elongation

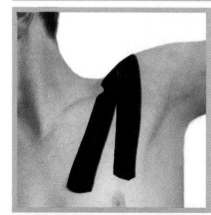

Serratus Anterior Assist

The serratus anterior is a muscle that is innervated by the long thoracic nerve. This nerve arises from the anterior nerve roots of the fifth, sixth and seventh cervical roots. As the serratus anterior contracts it causes the scapula to move anterior, holding it flat against the chest wall during protraction. Upward rotation of the scapula is provided by a force couple of the upper, middle, lower trapezius, and serratus anterior.

The alignment of the scapula at rest is in slight upward rotation with the inferior angle of the scapula further away from the spine. Children with serratus anterior weakness may exhibit medial winging of the scapula. In addition the scapula may be positioned in slight downward rotation with the inferior angle of the scapula closer to the spine. The rhomboids may be shortened and tight, and the lower trapezius fibers are overstretched and weak.

The clinical picture may present with the serratus anterior as either overstretched and weak or short and weak, resulting in poor scapula stability, medial winging of the scapula and inability to raise the arm properly. Therefore careful muscle examinations are important. Kinesio® Tape can be applied to stabilize the scapula on the rib cage to assist with active reach.

Serratus Anterior
Origin: 1-9th ribs
Insertion: Medial border of scapula
Action: Pulls the scapula anteriorly toward the ribs, abducts the scapula (protracts), acts as a force couple with the upper, middle and lower trapezius to upwardly rotate the scapula.

A 1.5 or 2 inch "Y" or fan tape (3 tails)

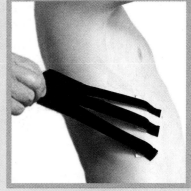

- Measure the "Y" tape or fan shape length from the anterior rib cage toward medial border of the scapula
- Cut the tape so 1/3 is an anchor and 2/3 are split into three tails
- Anchor the tails on ribs 4 to 6

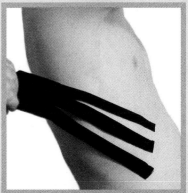

- Position arm in humeral flexion (90°-110°)
- Apply the tape with paper off tension to each of the tails, diagonally along the ribs, wrapping around the lateral border of the rib cage

- Continue to apply the tape with paper-off tension, moving toward the medial border of the scapula
- No tension is applied at the end of the tape

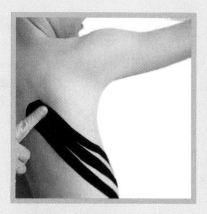

- Complete taping for the serratus anterior

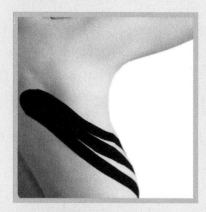

Alternate taping:

- Alternate taping for the serratus anterior can be done with an "I" strip, anchored at the origin of the serratus and applied toward the insertion
- Position arm in 90° to 110° humeral flexion
- Anchor the tape on ribs 4 to 6
- Apply the tape with paper-off tension diagonally along the ribs, wrapping around the lateral borders of the rib cage

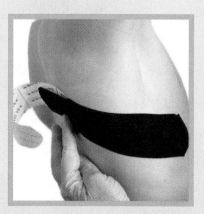

- Continue to apply the tape with paper-off tension, toward the medial border of the scapula
- No tension is applied at the end of the tape

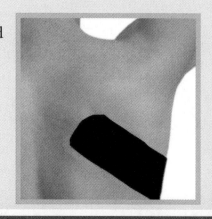

Shoulder External Rotation

The muscles which externally rotate the humerus consist of the infraspinatus and teres minor. The primary action is to stabilize the head of the humerus in the glenoid fossa and laterally rotate the shoulder joint. The supraspinatus assist with abduction of the shoulder joint and also stabilizes the head of the humerus during movement of this joint. The deltoid and supraspinatus work together to initiate abduction of the humerus.

Children with CNS dysfunction or muscular imbalance often present with difficulty actively moving the humerus into external rotation for reach. If the child is unable to actively externally rotate, this may limit the range of forearm supination with the elbow extended. In addition, limitation in lateral rotation may be caused by tightness in the following areas: anterior joint capsule, middle and inferior glenohumeral ligament, subscapularis, coracohumeral ligament, pectoralis, and anterior fascial restriction.

A 1.5 or 2 inch "I" tape

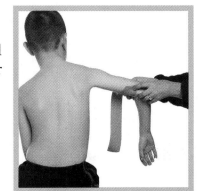

- Measure the tape length from the medial epicondyle, around the anterior surface of the humerus, and across the posterior deltoid and spine of the scapula toward the spine
- Place the arm into internal rotation, with the elbow flexed
- Anchor the tape at the medial epicondyle

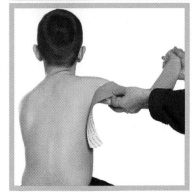

- Apply the tape with paper-off tension, wrapping it around the anterior surface of the humerus in an upward direction toward the posterior deltoid
- As tape is applied, gradually move the arm into external rotation

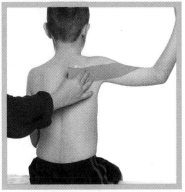

- Complete taping with the arm positioned in external rotation, while applying tape with paper-off tension across the spine of scapula
- No tension is applied at the end of the tape

Alternate taping:
- Position shoulder in neutral horizontal adduction (or less horizontal abduction), for less pull into shoulder external rotation
- Amount of horizontal abduction required may vary

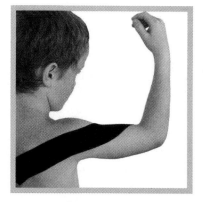

- Completed taping for shoulder external rotation

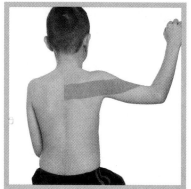

- Side view of completed taping for shoulder external rotation

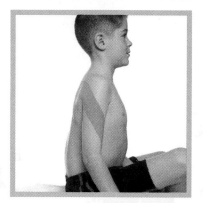

Deltoid Assist

Origin: Lateral clavicle, acromion, and spine of scapula
Insertion: Deltoid tuberosity of humerus
Action: The deltoid muscle is a bulky muscle that surrounds the shoulder girdle. It attaches on the spine of the scapula, acromion, and lateral third of the clavicle and inserts into the deltoid tuberosity on the humeral shaft. The middle deltoid assist with humeral abduction, the anterior fibers act in flexion and medial rotation and the posterior fibers act in extension and lateral rotation.

Weakness of the deltoid muscle may make lifting of the arm difficult. This is often seen in a child with a brachial plexus injury, spinal cord injury, CVA hemiplegia, or traumatic brain injury. The tape is applied from origin to insertion to assist with the movement for lifting the arm.

A 1.5 or 2 inch "Y" tape

- Measure from the acromion to the deltoid tuberosity with the arm resting at the side
- Anchor the tape at the acromion
- With the elbow and shoulder flexed, bring arm into horizontal adduction toward opposite shoulder
- Maintain posterior deltoid in elongated position
- Apply paper-off tension to the tape as it is applied along the posterior fibers of the deltoid
- No tension is applied at the end of the tape

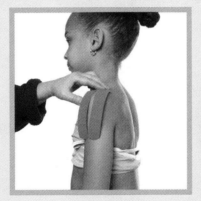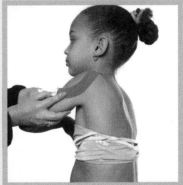

- Extend the humerus, elongating the anterior deltoid
- Apply tape with paper-off tension along the anterior fibers of the deltoid
- No tension is applied at the end of the tape

- Completed taping to facilitate deltoids

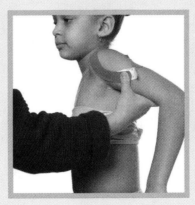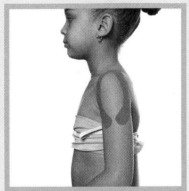

Alternate Deltoid: Relaxation

Overuse of the deltoid muscle can occur in a child with cerebral palsy or brachial plexus injury with a compensatory pattern of using humeral abduction and upper trapezius for lifting of the arm. The muscle can become painful from overuse or the muscle can become shortened from the compensatory movement. The taping technique of insertion to origin can assist in lengthening and relaxing the deltoid and releasing the fascia. This deltoid taping can be applied for an overused painful shoulder, and assist with seating the humeral head into the glenoid fossa.

A 1.5 or 2 inch "Y" tape

- Measure the tape from the deltoid tuberosity to the acromion
- Anchor the tape at the deltoid tuberosity

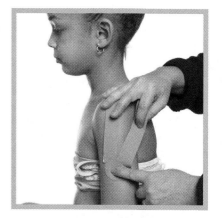

- With the elbow and humerus flexed, bring arm to horizontal adduction toward opposite shoulder
- Maintain posterior deltoid in elongated position
- Apply the tape with paper-off tension along the posterior fibers of the deltoid, toward the acromion
- No tension is applied at the end of the tape

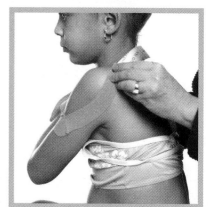

- Extend the humerus, elongating the anterior deltoid
- Apply tape with paper-off tension along the anterior fibers of the deltoid, toward the acromion
- No tension is applied at the end of the tape

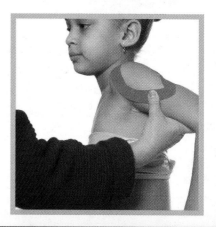

- Completed deltoid muscle taping, insertion to origin

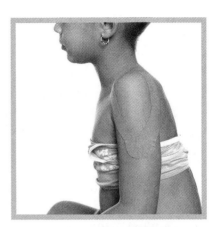

- Combined taping O to I, I to O
- Taping O to I and I to O together can provide greater stability of the shoulder girdle and assist with the movement of lifting and stabilizing the arm

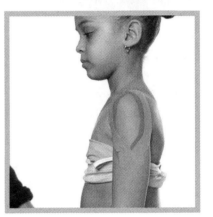

Elbow Taping

The elbow is a hinged joint that can functionally bring the child's hand to his mouth for feeding or assist for weight bearing while pushing off on a surface. The movement at the elbow is strongly linked to the kinematic chain of the trunk, scapula and shoulder. The placement of the child's hand is accomplished by the stability of the shoulder girdle, action of the elbow and orientation of the forearm.

The muscle activity of elbow extension is provided by the triceps and the anconeus. Basmajian, et al (1957) describe the muscle activity of elbow flexion as the following: the brachialis flexes at any rotational position of the forearm and at any speed; the biceps is active when the forearm is supinated when unloaded; the bicep is not active when the forearm is pronated unless it is loaded, as well as in a neutral rotation if a load is lifted; and the brachioradialis is active with a loaded forearm in a neutral rotation.

The alignment and active muscle control throughout the kinematic chain is crucial for efficient movement needed at the elbow. Taping proximally at the shoulder and trunk may need to be addressed, as well as the muscles of the elbow. Children with brachial plexus injury, orthopedic injury or CNS dysfunction may exhibit poor shoulder girdle stability, weak rotator cuff musculature, including weakness with elbow flexion or extension. In some cases, the pronated posture of the forearm may affect the child's ability to flex the elbow using the bicep muscles. The child may use a compensatory pattern of humeral abduction and elbow flexion with the forearm pronated. Children with CNS dysfunction may exhibit limited range of motion into elbow extension due to tightness and shortening of the elbow flexor muscles and/or over-lengthening of the triceps muscles with weakness into elbow extension. In the presence of severe abnormal tone and fixed contractures at the elbow, the child may initially require an aggressive treatment approach of splinting or positioning, serial casting, botulinum toxin and/ or medication to assist with relaxing the muscles. As the range and flexibility improves around the elbow joint, Kinesio® Taping can assist to relax the tight muscles and to assist the weakened muscles. In addition, a home program with positioning and ongoing strengthening program is critical to maintain the muscle balance.

1. Basmajian, JF and Latif A. (1957). Integrated actions and functions of the chief flexors of the elbow: A detailed electromyographic analysis. J Bone Jt. Surg. 39A: 1106-1118.

Biceps brachii
Origin: Short head arises from the coracoid process and the long head arises from the supraglenoid tubercle of the scapula.
Insertion: Tuberosity of the radius and aponeurosis of the biceps brachii (lacertus fibrosus).
Action: The biceps brachii muscle is the primary elbow flexor. It inserts on the radial tuberosity which also is an important supinator of the radius.

Elbow Flexion

Weakness of the biceps brachii muscle may make bringing the hand to the mouth or bringing objects toward the body difficult. This is often seen in a child with brachial plexus injury, spinal cord injury, CVA stroke, or traumatic brain injury. The child may compensate using humeral abduction and forearm pronation due to elbow flexion weakness.

Biceps Assist
A 1.5 or 2 inch "X" tape, a 1.5 or 2 inch "I" tape

- Measure from the supraglenoid tubercle and coracoid process to the proximal third of the supinated forearm with the elbow positioned in 30°-45° flexion

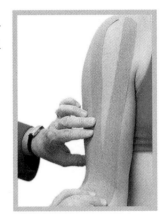

> **i** to assist the elbow into flexion the angle of the elbow joint determine the tension of the assist into flexion. Initially apply the tape with the elbow in 30°-45° flexion. The more the joint is flexed the greater the flexion assists; however observe for too much stress on the skin and tension on the muscle.

- Anchor the medial tail on the coracoid process and apply paper-off tension encircling the biceps toward the antecubital crease with the forearm in a supinated position.

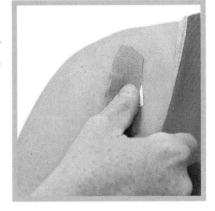

- Anchor the lateral tail of the tape at the supraglenoid tubercle and apply paper-off tension surrounding the biceps toward the antecubital crease

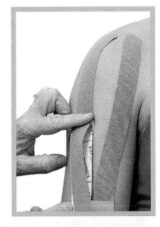

Upper Extremity

- Apply paper-off tension on the middle portion of the "X" with the elbow in 30° to 45° flexion
- The forearm is in a supinated position

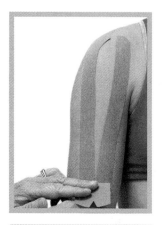

- Apply paper-off tension to the lateral and medial tails of the distal "X" at the proximal third of the forearm on the radius and ulna with the forearm supinated and elbow in flexion

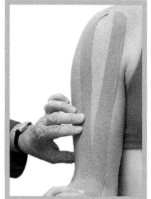

An additional piece of tape can be applied, origin to insertion, to provide more assist with flexion of the elbow
- Measure the "I" tape from the supraglenoid fossa to the proximal third of the supinated forearm with the elbow in a flexed position
- Anchor the tape at the supraglenoid fossa

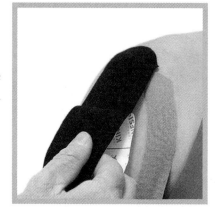

- Apply the tape with paper-off tension, extending the tape to the proximal third of the forearm
- No tension is applied at the end of the tape

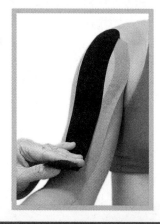

- Completed taping for biceps assist: origin to insertion

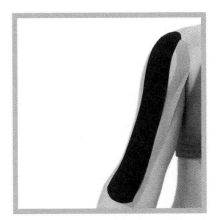

An alternative method of assisting the weak biceps can be applied using the functional assist technique.
- Anchor the tape proximally at the supraglenoid tubercle and at the proximal third of the forearm
- Leave a space between the proximal and distal anchor

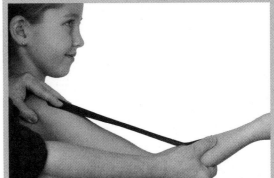

- Extend the elbow as you rub down the tape over the biceps

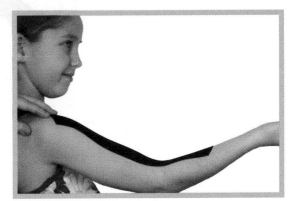

Biceps Brachii Relaxation

Tightness of the biceps brachii or shortening of this muscle can occur because of spasticity, postural fixation or compensatory patterns. This alternate taping technique of insertion to origin can assist to lengthen or relax the biceps brachii muscle.

A 1.5 or 2 inch "X" tape, a 1.5 or 2 inch "I" tape

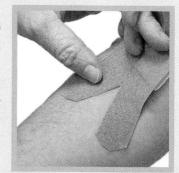

- Measure the tape from the proximal third of the forearm to the supraglenoid fossa with the elbow in extension and humerus in 30° extension.
- Anchor the tails of the tape at the proximal third of the forearm on the radius and ulna with the forearm supinated and elbow and humerus in extension
- Apply paper-off tension to the middle portion of the "X"

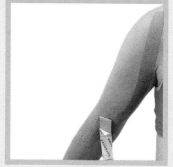

- With the elbow and the humerus extended, apply the medial tail with paper-off tension, encircling the biceps brachii, and moving toward the coracoid process
- No tension is applied at the end of the tape

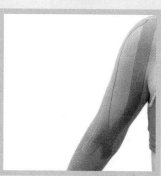

- Apply the lateral tail with paper-off tension, encircling the biceps brachii toward the supraglenoid tubercle
- No tension is applied at the end of the tape

An "I" tape, applied insertion to origin with the biceps in a lengthened position, may be used instead of the "Y" tape or in conjunction with the "Y" tape.

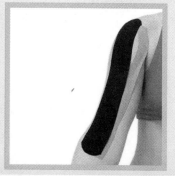

- Measure the "I" tape from the proximal third of the supinated forearm to the supraglenoid fossa with the elbow and humerus in an extended position
- Anchor the tape at the proximal third of the forearm
- Apply the tape with paper-off tension toward the supraglenoid fossa
- No tension is applied at the end of the tape
- Completed taping for bicep relaxation

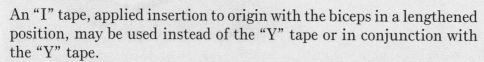

Triceps Assist

Triceps Brachii and Anconeus

Origin: Long head - infraglenoid tubercle, lateral head - posterior surface of humerus; medial head –medial and posterior surface of humerus
Insertion: Posterior surface of olecranon process of ulna and antebrachial fascia
Action: Primary elbow extensor

Elbow Extension:
Weakness of the tricep muscle may make extending the arm forward or overhead for reach difficult. This is often seen in a child with BPI, CP, CVA or TBI. The triceps brachii muscle is often in an over lengthened position and weak due to the flexed posture of the involved limb. Kinesio® Tape can be applied from origin to insertion to assist with the movement of straightening the elbow. It can also be applied as a biomechanical assist, limiting elbow flexion.

A 1.5 or 2 inch "I" tape

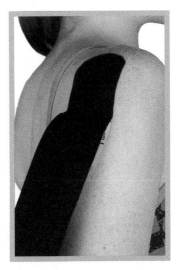

- Measure the "I" tape proximally from the posterior medial surface of the humerus to the proximal third of the forearm
- Anchor the tape at the posterior medial surface of the humerus

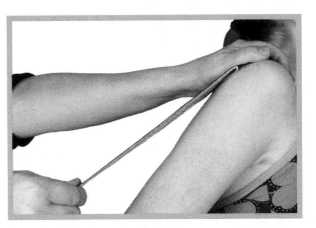

- Maintain the position of the elbow in slight flexion (15° - 20°), or fully extended
- Apply the tape with paper-off tension from the anchor, over the posterior surface of the olecranon, to the proximal third of the ulna
- No tension is applied at the end of the tape

- Completed taping for triceps assist

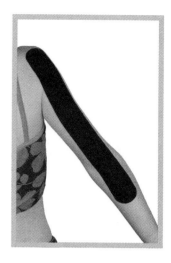

Alternate Triceps Assist
A 2 inch or 1.5 inch "Y" tape

- Position the elbow in slight flexion (15° - 20°) or fully extended
- Measure the tape length from the proximal posterior surface of the humerus, past the olecranon, to the proximal third of the posterior surface of the forearm
- Cut the tape so 2/3 is the "I" and 1/3 is the tail
- Anchor the tape at the infraglenoid tubercle (posterior proximal humerus)
- Apply the tape with paper-off tension along the posterior surface of the humerus, ending above the olecranon fossa

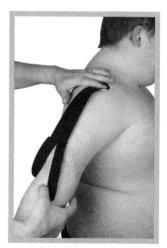

- Using paper-off tension, apply the medial tail of the "Y" tape around the medial epicondyle and encircle the elbow
- No tension is applied at the end of the tape

- Using paper-off tension, apply the lateral tail around the lateral epicondyle and encircle the elbow
- No tension is applied at the end of the tape
- Completed taping for triceps assist

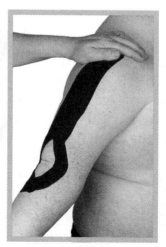
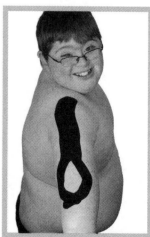

Lateral Epicondylitis

Lateral epicondylitis is commonly referred to as tennis elbow, however this condition is not exclusive to tennis players. It is an inflammatory condition of the extensor origin over the lateral epicondyle. It may be caused by a partial tear of the fibers of origin of the extensor muscles. The patient may be complaining of pain in the lateral aspect of the elbow. There may be localized pain or tenderness over the lateral epicondyle. This pain may be seen in the adolescent population with CNS disorder secondary to abnormal posturing of the forearm and wrist, with excessive pronation and wrist extension.

A 1.5 or 2 inch "Y" tape, a 2 inch "I" tape

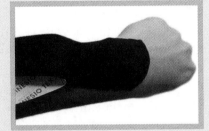

- Measure the tape length from the base of the 2nd and 3rd metacarpal to the lateral epicondyle
- Anchor the base of the "Y" at the 2nd and 3rd metacarpal, with the wrist in flexion

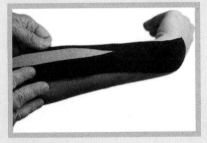

- Position the wrist in flexion, with forearm pronation, to elongate the extensors
- Apply the tails with paper-off tension, around the medial and lateral margins of the extensor muscles
- No tension is applied at the end of the tape as it surrounds the lateral epicondyle, ending just proximal to the lateral epicondyle

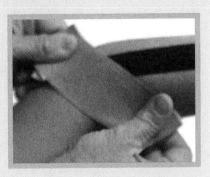

A Space Correction Technique is used for lifting fascia and soft tissue over the area of pain
- Tear the tape backing in the center and fold back the edges
- Apply over the area of localized pain, with full tension in the center of the tape
- No tension is applied at the ends of the tape

- The correctional tape assists with positioning the forearm in neutral and reduction of pain
- Completed taping for lateral epicondylitis

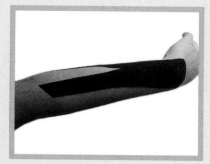

Alternate: space correction technique:
A 1.5 or 2 inch "I" tape

- With the elbow in slight flexion, anchor the "I" tape above the lateral epicondyle with no tension
- Apply the tape with moderate tension in a diagonal along the dorsal surface of the forearm, to form a spiral toward the volar surface of the mid-forearm

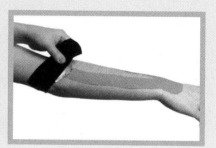

Forearm Supination Wrap

O: Lateral epicondyle of humerus and ulna crest
I: Lateral surface of the upper radius
A: Supinate forearm

The ability to combine movements of the forearm and wrist is essential for orienting the hand in the alignment needed to grasp an object for function such as, drinking from a cup, writing, or feeding. The abnormal tone of the pronator muscles or muscle imbalance can position the forearm into pronation. The ability for the child to orient the hand for function is diminished due to the inability to rotate the forearm into supination. The pronated forearm biomechanically places the hand in poor alignment i.e. wrist flexion, ulnar deviation and thumb adduction or flexion. The control of both pronation and supination is required; however supination can be limited by the spasticity of the pronator muscles and the influence of the alignment of the shoulder girdle.

A 1.5 or 2 inch "I" tape

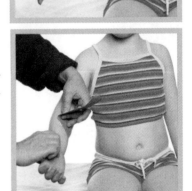

- Measure the tape length from the 2nd and 3rd metacarpals on the dorsum of hand toward the ulna, wrapping around the mid-forearm on the volar side, to the lateral epicondyle
- Apply the anchor of tape on the dorsum of the 2nd and 3rd metacarpals
- Position the arm in pronation and wrist flexion
- As the forearm is moved into supination, apply the tape with paper-off tension, diagonally toward the mid-forearm

- Continue to gradually supinate the forearm, while applying tape with paper-off tension on the volar surface, diagonally toward the radius and the lateral epicondyle

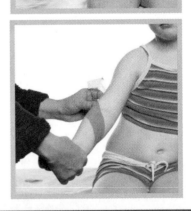

- Complete taping with the forearm in supination
- Adhere the tape near lateral epicondyle
- No tension is applied at the end of the tape

Upper Extremity

Alternate Taping for Forearm Supination Assist

This technique can be used to provide subtle input to facilitate supination. It can be used to assist a child with mild involvement to position the forearm in neutral and with movement into supination.

A 1.5 or 2 inch "I" tape

- Measure from the lateral epicondyle to the radial styloid process
- Anchor the tape at the lateral epicondyle

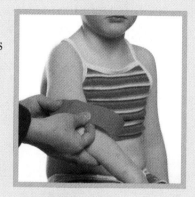

- Position the forearm in neutral alignment
- Apply the tape with minimal tension (15-20 %) toward the radial styloid process

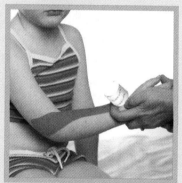

- Anchor the tape on the midforearm
- The tape can extend toward distal radius with no tension at the end

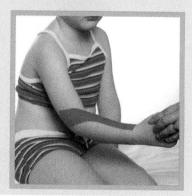

Alternate Taping for Forearm Supination: Fascial Correction

Prior to applying the Kinesio® Tape, it is important to assess the restriction in the forearm and provide manual therapy. Techniques include joint mobilization, myofascial release or modalities to improve the range and active movement. This taping technique may be applied to any area that has fascial restrictions. Measure and apply the tape accordingly.

A 1.5 or 2 inch "Y" tape

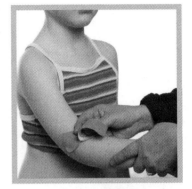

- Measure from lateral epicondyle in a diagonal to the proximal third forearm on the volar surface
- Cut the tape 50-50 (half anchor and half tails) for the "Y"
- Anchor the tape at the lateral epicondyle

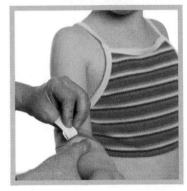

- Use a "jiggle" technique
- Hold onto each tail while slowly jiggling rapidly from side to side with paper-off tension, to gather the fascia

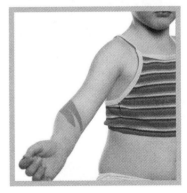

- The completed taping for fascial correction for supination

Forearm Pronation Assist

Pronator Teres

Origin: Medial epicondyle
 Insertion: Lateral surface of the radius
Action: Pronates the forearm

A 1.5 inch or 2 inch "I" tape

- Measure the tape length from the medial epicondyle to the lateral surface of the radius
- Anchor the tape at the medial epicondyle, with the forearm in a supinated position

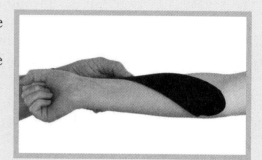

- Ask patient to pronate forearm, or move forearm into pronation during tape application
- Apply the tape with paper-off tension on a diagonal, toward the lateral third of the radius
- No tension is applied at the end of the tape

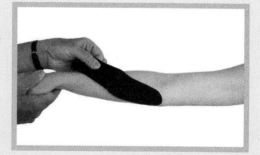

- Completed taping to facilitate forearm pronation

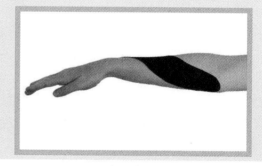

Carpal Tunnel Syndrome

Carpal tunnel syndrome is a compression neuropathy of the median nerve at the wrist. The carpal tunnel is formed by the articulated carpal bones and roofed by the transverse carpal ligament. The tunnel contains all the flexor tendons and the median nerve passing through the wrist into the palm. The child or adolescent can complain of numbness or tingling of the first three fingers and pain at the wrist. The nerve can become ischemic from repetitive wrist extension with finger flexion as seen with children with dystonic movements.

Cailliet R. (1982). Hand Pain and Impairment. Philadelphia: F.A. Davis Company.

A 1.5 or 2 inch "X" tape

- Measure from the thenar and hypothenar eminence proximally to the lateral epicondyle
- Cut "X" with two tails long and two tails short
- Tear the middle portion of the "X" tape
- Position the wrist in slight extension, palm side up, and put moderate tension to the tape as it is applied over the wrist and distal forearm

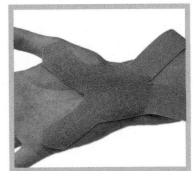

- Maintain the wrist in slight extension
- Apply one distal tail to the thenar eminence and the other tail to the hypothenar eminence with paper-off tension

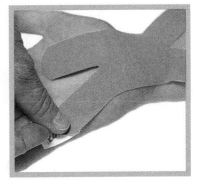

- Apply the proximal tails of the "X" tape on the forearm in the direction of the medial epicondyle and lateral epicondyle with paper-off tension

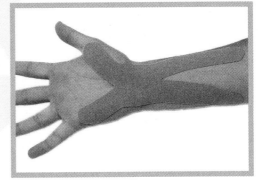

- Cut a space correction "I" tape
- Measure "I" tape around the wrist on the dorsal surface, from the radial to the ulnar side
- Tear "I" tape backing in the middle and fold back the edges
- Position the wrist in neutral
- Take moderate tension from the center of tape and apply on the dorsum of the wrist
- Apply the ends toward the volar side of the wrist with no tension

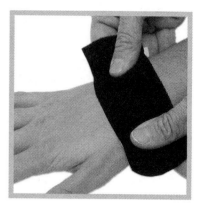

ℹ Edges should just overlap palmar taping. Do not wrap correction tape circumferentially around the wrist.

- Completed taping for carpal tunnel syndrome

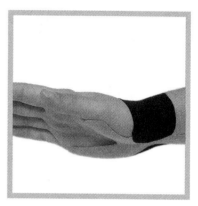

Alternate Taping for Carpal Tunnel Syndrome: Space Correction Technique

A 1.5 or 2 inch "I" tape

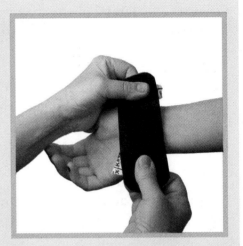

- Measure "I" tape on the volar surface of the wrist, starting from thumb side and extending to the little finger
- Tear the tape in the center and fold back the backing
- Position the wrist in slight extension
- Take moderate to full tension from the middle of tape and apply on the volar surface of the wrist

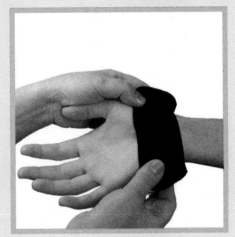

- No tension is applied at the ends
- Do not wrap circumferentially around the wrist

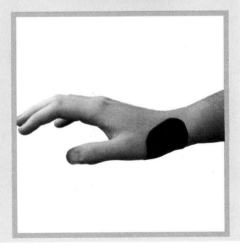

- Completed taping for carpal tunnel syndrome

Wrist Extension Assist

Extensor carpi radialis longus
Origin: lateral epicondyle and supracondylar ridge of the humerus
Insertion: Base of 2nd metacarpal

Extensor carpi radialis brevis
Origin: Lateral epicondyle of humerus
Insertion: Base of 3rd metacarpal

Action: Extends and abducts the wrist

Extensor carpi ulnaris
Origin: Lateral epicondyle of humerus and posterior border of ulna
Insertion: Base of 5th metacarpal

Action: Ulna adduction and wrist extension

Functional Correction Technique

A 1.5 or 2 inch "I" tape

- Measure tape length from the metacarpals to the lateral epicondyle
- Extend the wrist
- Apply the anchor on the dorsum of the hand, over the metacarpals

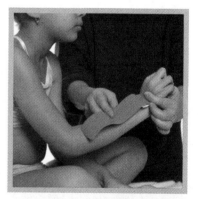

- Maintain the wrist in extension
- Apply the proximal anchor of tape on the lateral epicondyle
- Leave a space between the tape and forearm
- Area of greater tension may be targeted by anchoring proximal to the lateral epicondyle, with more tension to tape on specific area over wrist

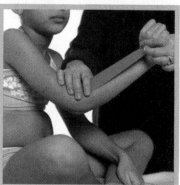

- Flex the wrist as you rub the tape down over dorsum of the forearm

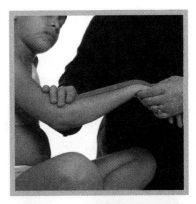

- The tape will assist with active wrist extension
- Completed taping to facilitate wrist extension

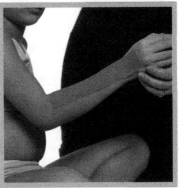

Alternate Technique: Buttonhole Wrist Extension Assist

The buttonhole technique provides proprioceptive input into the palm of the hand as well as assisting with wrist extension

A 1.5 or 2 inch "I" tape

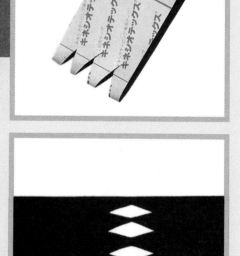

- Tape will extend from the palmar surface of the hand, through the fingers to the lateral elbow
- Measure tape length from the dorsal surface of the hand to the lateral epicondyle, and add length of palmar surface of the hand

> **i** If the palmar portion of the tape does not stay on, the tape can be extended past the wrist

- Fold the distal third of the tape measuring the area of the palmar surface to be taped
- Cut three triangular shapes for fingers to be placed, which will become diamond-shaped when unfolded

- Open the tape and gently tear the backing from the areas cut for the fingers
- Pull the backing off on both sides of the diamonds and fold back

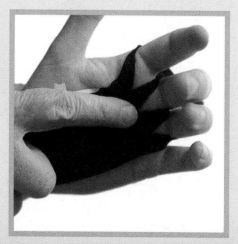

- Gently place the index, middle and ring finger through the holes
- Avoid jamming or applying too much pressure in between the fingers

Upper Extremity

- Apply paper-off tension to tape on the palmar surface of the hand
- Anchor dorsal side of tape at the metacarpals

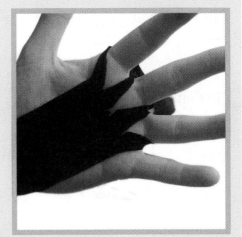

- Extend the wrist
- Apply the proximal anchor on the forearm toward the lateral epicondyle
- An area of greater tension may be created by anchoring the tape midforearm which places more tension over the wrist
- Leave a space between the tape and forearm, as previously described in the functional correction technique for wrist extension
- Flex the wrist as you rub down over dorsum of the wrist
- Rub tape to adhere

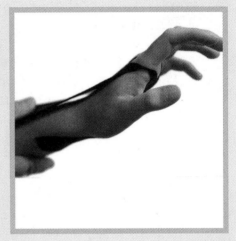

- Completed buttonhole wrist extension taping technique

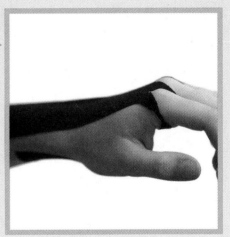

Buttonhole Technique for Edema

Edema is swelling caused by fluid retention. Swelling can occur if the body is not circulating fluid well. It is often seen after hand surgery, as well as in sub-acute or chronic stroke injury or trauma. The skin may be taut and shiny, with uniform swelling in the forearm and hand. Kinesio® Taping Method, along with traditional treatment techniques of manual edema mobilization or myofascial release, is helpful in removing the congested lymph fluid from the area. Providing the low stretch from the Kinesio® Tape can stimulate the lymphatic system.

A 1.5 or 2 inch "I" tape with diamond-shaped cutouts for fingers

- Measure from the metacarpophalangeal (MCP) joints of the volar surface of the hand to the proximal half of the forearm, and equal distance on the dorsal surface
- Fold the tape in half and cut three triangular shapes for the fingers to be placed
- These become diamond-shaped openings in the tape, wide enough for the fingers to fit through

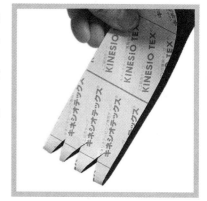

- Tear the tape at the buttonhole area and pull the paper off on both sides, slowly folding back
- Gently place the fingers through the buttonholes and lay tape down in the web space of the fingers
- Do not put any tension on the tape as it is laid down between the fingers

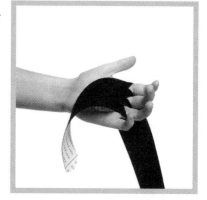

- Place the wrist in extension
- Apply the tape with paper-off tension in the palm

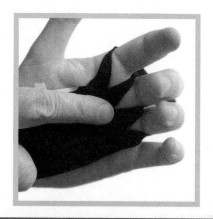

- Apply the tape with paper-off tension along the volar surface of the forearm
- No tension is applied at the end of the tape

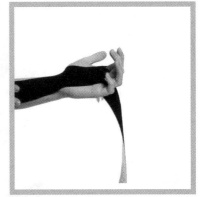

- Place the wrist in flexion
- Apply the tape with paper-off tension along the dorsal surface of the forearm
- No tension is applied at the end of the tape

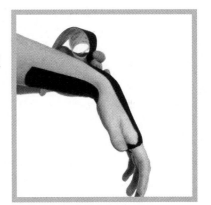

- Top view of buttonhole for edema

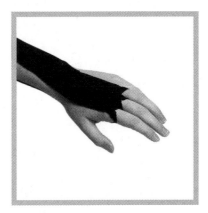

Wrist Radial Deviation

This is a functional correction technique to assist positioning the wrist in midline position. In children with CNS dysfunction or brachial plexus injuries, the wrist may be ulnarly deviated due to muscle imbalance or CNS involvement.

A 1 inch or ½ inch "I" tape

- Measure the tape length from the metacarpophalangeal (MCP) joint of the thumb to the distal third of the radius
- Position the hand in radial deviation
- Anchor the tape at MCP joint of the thumb

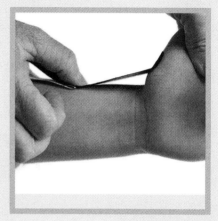

- Anchor the other end of the tape at mid-forearm, on the radial surface
- Maintain the wrist in radial deviation
- Leave a space between the tape and forearm

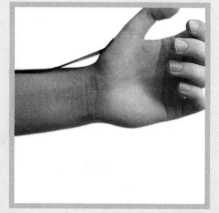

- Ulnarly deviate the wrist as you rub tape over the radial surface of forearm
- Completed taping for radial deviation

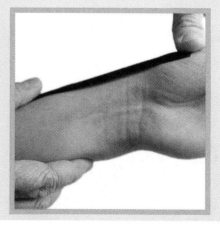

De Quervain's Tenosynovitis

De Quervain's is a constriction of the abductor pollicis longus and extensor pollicis brevis tendons of the thumb at the wrist. Repetitive movement of the tendons of the thumb may cause inflammation of the tendon sheaths and cause pain. The tenosynovitis may cause pain along the lateral aspect of the distal end of the radius. There may be swelling and inflammation along the tendons and tenderness on palpation. Taping the thumb into neutral alignment and placing a corrective strip on the lateral distal border of the radius where the tendons pass under the extensor retinaculum relieves the pain.

A 1 inch or ½ inch "I" tape, a 1 inch or ½ inch "X" tape

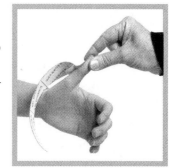

- Measure from the interphalangeal (IP) joint of the thumb to the mid-forearm along the radius
- Anchor the tape just distal to IP joint of thumb, with the elbow flexed and the wrist in a neutral position

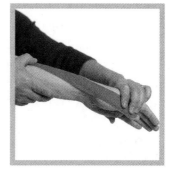

- Flex and ulnarly deviate the wrist as tolerated
- Position the thumb in flexion and apply paper off tension along extensor surface of forearm
- No tension is applied at the end of the tape

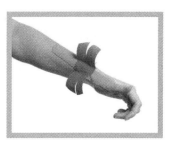

- A 1 inch or ½ inch "X" correction tape is then applied
- Measure the correction tape from the interosseus border on the dorsal and volar side of the forearm
- Tear the tape backing in the center and fold back edges
- Apply moderate to full stretch to the center of the tape, as it is applied in anatomical snuffbox region or over the area of pain

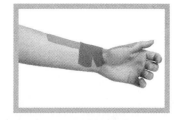

Correction tape
- Apply the tails with no tension, to distribute force

Thumb Taping

There are eight muscles that insert on the thumb. Four of the eight muscles are the extrinsic muscles that cross the wrist and four are the intrinsic muscles of the thumb. Weakness or muscle imbalance of the thumb at the metacarpophalangeal (MCP) joint has a significant effect on the function and fine motor skills of grasping between the thumb and the digits. Opposition is essential for grasping or prehensile movements, which require reciprocal movements of both the thumb and digits. Napier describes the abductor pollicis brevis as the muscle responsible for positioning the thumb into abduction and rotation at the MCP joint. The ability to abduct and rotate the thumb takes place at both the MCP and carpometacarpal (CMC) joint. Without activity of the abductor polis brevis, tip to tip prehension of the thumb and digits cannot be achieved.

Weathersby et al evaluated the kinesiology of the thumb muscles. Electromyography was used to study the movement of the eight muscles of the thumb in ten test motions. The study found that six muscles were involved in five or more movements, and seven of the motions required contraction of five or more muscles to produce smooth, even, isotonic movement.

Children who present with increased spasticity or stiffness often times demonstrates tightness into flexion and adduction. The muscle imbalance prevents the thumb from actively extending or abducting at the MCP and interphalangeal (IP) joint. There is tightness in the thenar eminence and the child often has difficulty with palmar expansion. The ability to extend the thumb is often impaired, and there may be hyperextension of the IP or MCP joint with hypermobility of the MCP joint. Prior to Kinesio® Taping, it is important for the practitioner to observe isolated movements of the thumb, if present. The co-contraction of the muscles of the thumb demonstrates a delicate balance between the extrinsic and intrinsic muscles required for function. The inter-relationship of the thumb muscles must be considered when evaluating the muscle action and alignment for taping.

Napier JP. 1952. The attachments and function of the abductor pollicis brevis. Journal of Anatomy. 86:335-341.

Weathersby HT, Sutton LR, and Krusen UL. 1963. The kinesiology of muscles of the thumb: An electomyographic study. Archives of Physical Medicine and Rehabilitation. June, 321-326.

Thumb Extension Assist

Extensor Pollicis Longus
Origin: Ulna and interosseous membrane- middle 1/3
Insertion: Base of distal phalanx of thumb
Action: Extension of IP joint of thumb

Extensor Pollicis Brevis
Origin: Radius and interosseous membrane
Insertion: Base of proximal phalanx MCP
Action: Extension of MCP joint

A 1 inch or ½ inch "I" tape

- Measure the tape length from the interphalangeal (IP) joint of the thumb to distal third of the forearm
- Position the thumb into extension
- Anchor the tape at the thumb IP joint

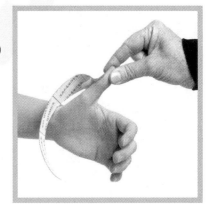

- Maintain the thumb in extension
- Apply proximal anchor of tape to middle third of interosseous membrane, on dorsal surface of forearm
- Leave a space between the tape and forearm

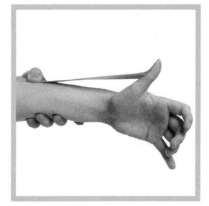

- Flex the thumb as you rub down the tape over the thumb and the dorsum of the forearm

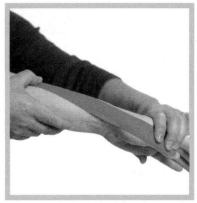

Thumb Metacarpophalangeal Stability Taping

Combined MCP stability taping and functional correction tape for thumb extension
A ½ inch or ¼ inch "I" tape

- For metacarpophalangeal (MCP) joint instability, place an "I" tape to support the joint
- Measure an "I" strip around the thumb
- Maintain slight flexion at the MCP joint
- Tear the tape in the middle and use downward pressure with the MCP joint in flexion
- No tension at the ends of tape and wrap around the joint

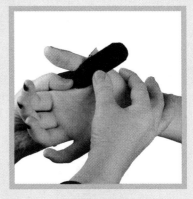

i Do not restrict circulation with the taping technique

- Completed taping for thumb extension and stabilization of the MCP joint

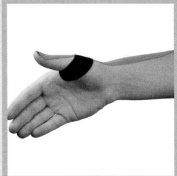

i For a thumb that exhibits increased spasticity, dystonia, or abnormal tone, extra support may be required to maintain alignment and stability at the MCP joint.

- For extra support, place an "I" tape using rigid tape, such as Leukotape, to support the joint
- Measure an "I" strip around the thumb
- Maintain slight flexion at the MCP joint
- Apply the middle of the tape and wrap each end around the thumb
- Do not apply stretch to the rigid tape

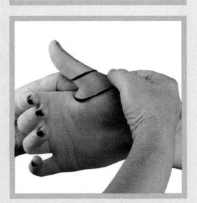

i Do not restrict circulation with the taping technique

Thenar Eminence Taping

This taping technique can assist with decreasing the tightness in the thenar eminence and to assist with opening of the hand for weight bearing, and to improve palmar expansion. The thenar eminence consists of the flexor pollicis brevis, abductor pollicis brevis, and opponens pollicis.

A ½ inch or ¼ inch "I" tape

- Measure from the trapezium, which is distal to the carpometacarpal (CMC) joint, along the thenar eminence up through the web space, and back around to the dorsal side -connecting to the beginning of the tape

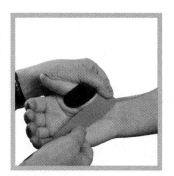

- Fully expand the palm and thenar eminence
- Anchor the tape at the trapezium, which is distal to the CMC joint
- Use paper-off tension on the tape and place downward pressure into the thenar eminence while applying the tape

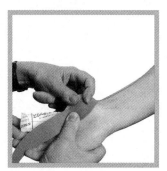

- Continue to use paper-off tension up through the web space and on the dorsum of the hand back to the CMC joint

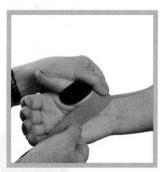

- Completed thenar eminence taping

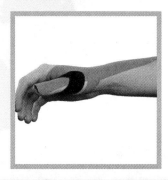

Combination Palmar Taping: in preparation for weight bearing

Combining the thenar eminence taping with the hypothenar eminence taping can assist with opening the hand for weight bearing, and decreasing tightness in the palm. The hypothenar eminence consists of the flexor digiti minimi brevis, abductor digiti minimi, and opponens digiti minimi.

Technique 1
A ½ inch or ¼ inch "I" tape

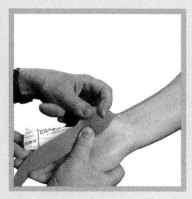

- Measure from the trapezium, which is distal to the carpometacarpal (CMC) joint, along the thenar eminence up through the web space, and back around to the dorsal side connecting to the beginning of the tape

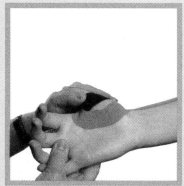

- Fully expand the palm and thenar eminence
- Anchor the tape at the trapezium, which is distal to the CMC joint
- Use paper-off tension on the tape and place downward pressure into the thenar eminence while applying the tape

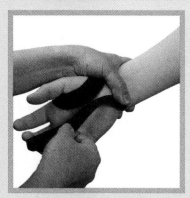

- Measure from the hamate (carpal bone) along the hypothenar eminence, and back around the dorsal side of the hand connecting to the beginning of the tape
- Fully expand the hypothenar eminence

- Anchor the tape at the hamate
- Use paper off tension of the tape and place downward pressure into the hypothenar eminence while applying the tape
- Continue to use paper off tension on the dorsum of the hand back toward the hamate

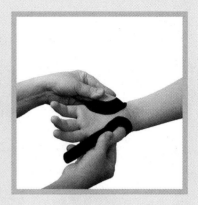

- Completed thenar and hypothenar eminence taping

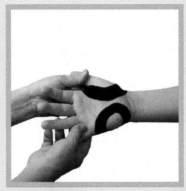

Palmar View

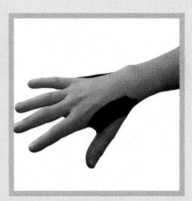

Dorsal View

Technique 2
Two ½ inch or ¼ inch "Y" tapes

- Measure tape length to extend from dorsal hand acrss thenar eminence
- Anchor tape at dorsum of the hand between the web space and the wrist

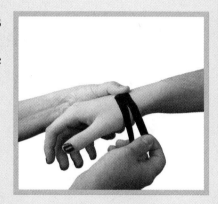

- Use minimal tension on the tape and place downward pressure into the thenar eminence while applying the tape one tail at a time

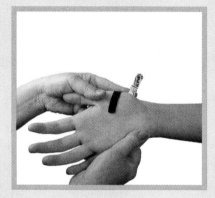

- Completed thenar side

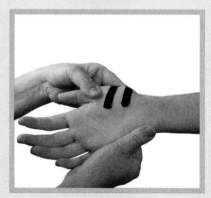

- Measure tape length to extend from dorsal hand across hypothenar eminence
- Anchor tape at dorsum of the hand between the 5th MCP and the wrist

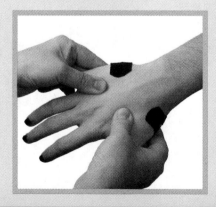

Upper Extremity

- Use minimal tension on the tape and place downward pressure into the hypothenar eminence while applying the tape one tail at a time

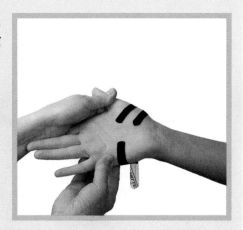

- Completed combination palmar taping

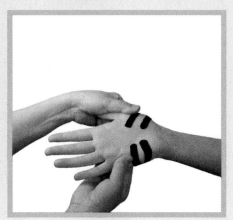

Finger Extension Assist

Extensor Digitorum

Origin: Lateral epicondyle of the humerus
Insertion: Distal phalanges of the digits (II-V)
Action: Extend and spread fingers (extends IP joint II-V, MCP joint and wrist joint)

For children with neurological disorders such as CP, TBI and CVA the ability to achieve full expansion of an open hand may be difficult due to increased tightness or spasticity of the wrist and fingers. This is because the digits may be dominated by marked flexion with a tightly fisted hand. Often times the child will release an object by flexing the wrist which biomechanically will extend the fingers. This is often seen with children using a compensatory tenodesis grasp and release pattern.

It is important to relax and stretch the tightness at the thenar and hypothenar eminence. By applying the various techniques such as neurodevelopmental treatment, myofascial release, joint mobilization, weight bearing etc., this may inhibit the abnormal tone and assist with promoting better alignment of the wrist and hand.

A neutral or slightly extended wrist, with a balance between the long finger flexors and the finger extensors will allow for stronger grip strength and functional prehension. It is important to evaluate the child's basic grip, position of the wrist and the ability to relax the grip to adequately extend the fingers. Kinesio® tape for active release will assist with the extension of the fingers; however it will take time, practice and repetition.

A 1.5 or 2 inch fan-shaped tape

- Measure the "I" portion of the tape from the lateral epicondyle to the wrist and the fan (4 strips) from the wrist to the nail bed of fingers 2-5

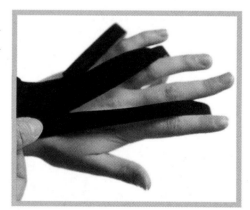

- Position the wrist in about 20° extension, with the fingers in extension
- Anchor the tape at the lateral epicondyle
- Apply the "I" portion of the tape with paper-off tension from the lateral epicondyle to the distal wrist, with the wrist in an extended position

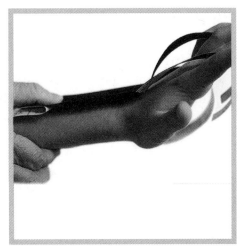

- Apply each tail with paper-off tension, from the carpals to the nail beds of fingers 2-5, with fingers in extension
- No tension is applied at the end of the tape

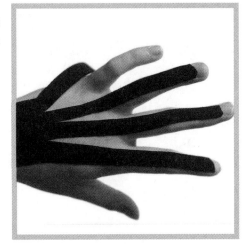

- Completed taping to facilitate finger extension

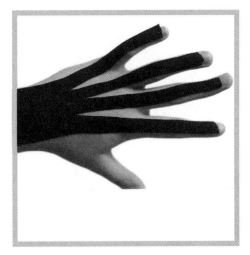

Palmar Stability

Manipulation is the ability to position the fingers and thumb to handle objects. Children acquire and refine these skills throughout their development. Precision handling and manipulation developed with the thumb in opposition and the fingertips on the object. Throughout the child's development there is a gradual refinement of movements.

Muscles used during object manipulation involve the intrinsic musculature of the hand. The intrinsics include the interossei, lumbricales, adductor pollicis and the thenar triad muscles of the thumb. In 1970, Long described the flexor pollicis brevis, opponens pollicis and abductor pollicis brevis as the thenar triad; which assist in the maintenance of the web space.

Children with musculoskeletal weakness of the hand or central nervous system dysfunction often present difficulties with fine motor prehension. The pattern most often used is mass grasp and release with poor thumb-finger opposition and decrease web space. Taping for palmar stability provides the proprioceptive input of stabilizing and facilitating fine finger movements. This taping technique also supports the web space. For extremely weak hands or wrist, a lumbricale splint or wrist splint may be applied in addition to the taping to strengthen the muscles needed for prehension.

Long, C., et al. (1970) Intrinsic-extrinsic muscle control of the hand in power grip and precision handling. The J of Bone & Joint Surg, 52-A, (5), 853-867.

Palmar Stability
A technique to improve fine motor skills for prehension

A 1 inch or 1.5 inch "Y" tape

- Measure the tape length from the palm through the web space, to third metacarpal
- The tape is a "Y" cut, with fifty percent anchor and fifty percent tails
- Position hand in neutral deviation; wrist in 20° extension

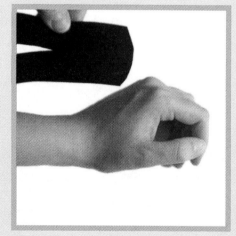

- Anchor the tape within palmer arch
- Tape is applied with paper-off tension through web space
- Tape may be extended to the base of the palm if it tends to peel off easily

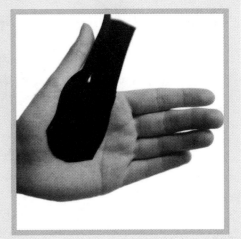

- Apply tails over dorsum of hand with paper-off tension in a diagonal direction
- No tension is applied at end of the tape
- This taping will support the palmar arch and web space

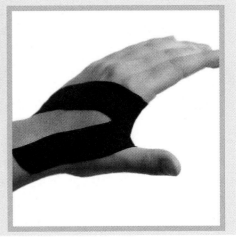

Wrist Radial Digital Grasp

Children with CNS or developmental delay may have difficulty with differentiation of the hand between the use of the ulnar and radial side. The radial digital grasp uses an opposed thumb and fingertips. The ring and little finger stabilizes the ulnar side of the hand. The radial palmar grasp develops from seven to nine months and matures into a radial digital grasp. From ten to twelve months the thumb opposes the index finger in a precise pincer grasp. The radial portion of the hand is used with the ulnar side of the fingers flexed for stabilizing the hand. The use of the radial-ulnar dissociation is critical when developing in-hand manipulation skills with the ability to stabilize the object within the child's hand. Children require adequate grasp patterns to facilitate the development of in-hand manipulation skills.

In-hand manipulation requires the use of both stability and mobility of the joints with control by the intrinsic musculature of the hand. Fine motor prehension skills require careful assessments of the child's abilities, limitations, and factors that contribute to the fine motor problems. Fine motor intervention must be balanced with adjunctive treatment. The child's active participation and repetition of actions is crucial for developing fine motor skills.

Case-Smith J and Pehoski C. 1992. Development of Hand Skills in the Child. Rockville,MD: The American Occupational Therapy Association, Inc.

Henderson A, and Pehoski C. 1995. Hand Function in the Child- Foundation for Remediation. St. Louis, MO: Mosby-Year Book, Inc.

Two ½ inch or ¼ inch "I" tapes

- Apply the palmar stability tape prior to taping the hand for radial digital grasp

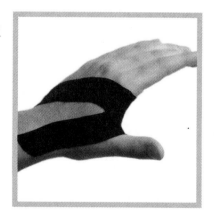

- Measure distance from wrist to distal interphalangeal joint (DIP) of middle finger for tape length of first piece of tape
- Measure distance from thumb interphalangeal joint (IP) to base of thenar eminence (trapezium) and continuing to interphalangeal joint (DIP) of first finger, for tape length of second piece of tape
- Maintain the hand fully open
- Apply the "I" tape along the longitudinal arch of the middle finger over the palmar stability tape
- Anchor the tape at the capitate, just distal to the wrist

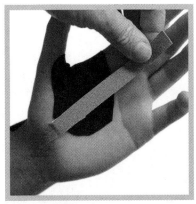

- Apply the tape with paper-off tension to the DIP joint, leaving the fingertip exposed for tactile input

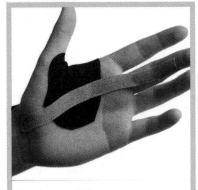

- Maintain the hand in a fully open position
- Tear the second "I" strip of tape about 1/3 of the length (measure from the trapezium to the IP joint of the thumb) and anchor the tape at the trapezium

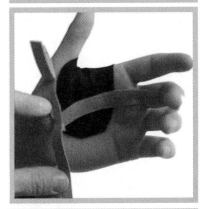

- Apply the tape with paper-off tension up toward the IP joint of the thumb, leaving the fingertip exposed for tactile input
- Continue by applying the other end of the tape, with paper-off tension, up to the DIP joint of the index finger leaving the fingertip exposed
- Completed taping for the facilitation of radial digital grasp

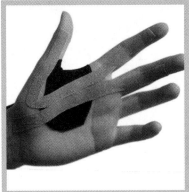

The oblique arch links the thumb to each fingertip for opposition

This tape is often worn just for a treatment session, or while working on handwriting skills or fine motor manipulation.

Jammed Finger

A jammed finger can occur from contact sports such as basketball, baseball, football or any type of activities that "jammed" the finger on the tip. The child typically sustains a blow to the finger combined with hyperextension and swelling of the proximal interphalangeal (PIP) joint occurs. To decrease the swelling, immediately apply ice and elevate the finger.

Careful assessment is critical to rule out fracture of the growth plate, a dislocation, integrity of the neurovascular status or collateral ligament injury. However an x-ray may be necessary to determine the status of the growth plate. Observe active finger movement in flexion and extension. The loss of finger extension may indicate a central slip injury. If there is no fracture or dislocation the jammed finger should heal completely.

Two ½ inch or ¼ inch "I" tapes, four ¼ inch "I" tapes

- Apply "I" strips on dorsal or volar surface of injured joint, using moderate tension limiting position of injury (flexion or extension)

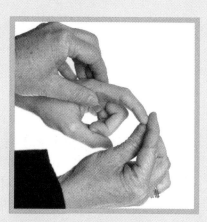

- Cut 2 small strips of tape lengthwise

- Apply strips using moderate to maximal tension in the center of the tape, with no tension on the ends

- These strips assist to stabilize the injured joint, as well as to assist in decreasing edema

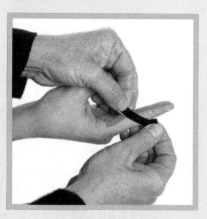

- Support the joint with an "X" tape over medial and lateral joint, with moderate to maximal tension on the center of the tape

- No tension at the ends of the tape

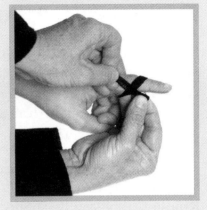

- A strip of tape may be added proximal and distal to the PIP joint using <u>no tension</u> to assist with holding the other pieces of tape in place

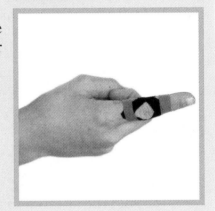

- <u>Do not</u> wrap completely around the finger with the added strips

- Be aware of any tightness, change in circulation or complaints of numbness in the finger after the tape has been applied

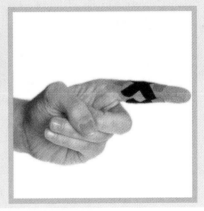

Upper Extremity Postural Alignment

A child with CNS dysfunction or peripheral nerve injury may present with compensatory or associated patterns of movement and fascial restriction. Upper extremity concerns may include synergistic movement patterns (i.e. flexor or extensor), soft tissue restrictions, decreased proprioceptive input with an altered sense of postural midline, and subsequent functional disuse. Musculoskeletal asymmetries can occur from abnormal tone or stiffness, muscle imbalances, including unopposed muscle firing of the antagonist, and compensatory patterns. Evaluation of the child must include careful assessment of the movement patterns. It is important to assess the joint end-feel and quality of the muscle and tissue, as well.

Kinesio® Tape can be applied to position the upper extremity in more optimal alignment for movement. The determination of appropriate taping techniques will rely on a proper evaluation of the upper extremity, skeletal alignment and muscle imbalances. Poor upper extremity positioning can bind down the fascia, resulting in inefficient movement, as well as postural malalignment. Kinesio® Taping can assist to realign the child's upper extremity.

Technique 1: (Extended Reach)
A 1.5 or 2 inch "I" or "Y" tape

- Measure the length of the tape from the wrist, wrapping around the forearm, to the triceps, across the spine of the scapula to the spine
- Anchor the tape at the dorsal wrist (can use "buttonhole" cut technique for wrist extension and palmar input)
- Position the wrist into extension
- Place second anchor on the distal third of the forearm, leaving space in between the tape and the hand

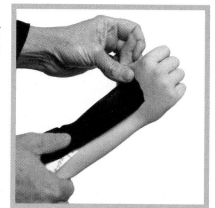

- Place the wrist into flexion while holding the anchors to stabilize the tape and gently rub the tape proximal to distal
- This functional assist focuses the tension on the wrist area, between the anchors, to provide optimal support to the wrist extensors

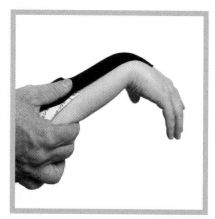

- Wrap the tape around the forearm with paper-off tension, as the forearm is gradually supinated

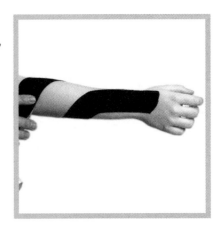

- Slightly flex or fully extend the elbow and continue taping along the triceps

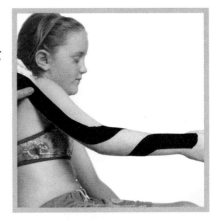

- Position the arm forward into horizontal adduction
- Apply the superior tail along the spine of the scapula

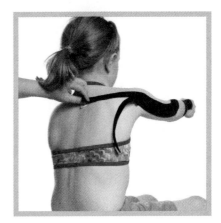

- Position the arm in humeral flexion

- Apply the posterior tail along the lateral side of rib cage towards its origin*

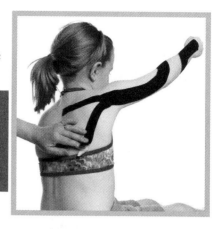

> ℹ *The posterior tail can be cut longer to apply toward the origin of the latissimus dorsi (the thoracolumbar aponeurosis, iliac crest and sacrum) depending on the tightness of the latissimus dorsi

- Completed taping for postural alignment
- This taping technique can assist the child with functional synergies, linking groups of muscles with the proprioceptive input and sensation from the Kinesio® tape to improve active reach with optimal alignment

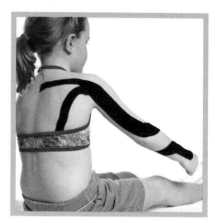

- Measure the length of the tape from the wrist, wrapping to the volar surface of the forearm, toward the origin of the biceps
- Anchor the tape at the dorsal wrist (can use "buttonhole" cut technique for wrist extension and palmar input)
- Position the wrist into extension
- Place second anchor on the distal third of the forearm, leaving space in between tape and the hand

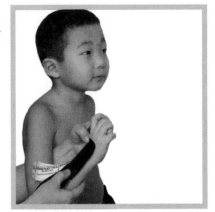

- Place the wrist into flexion while holding the anchors to stabilize the tape and gently rub the tape proximal to distal
- This functional assist focuses the tension on the wrist area, between the anchors, to provide optimal support to the wrist extensors

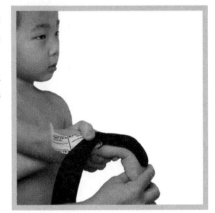

- Wrap the tape around the forearm with paper-off tension, as the forearm is gradually supinated

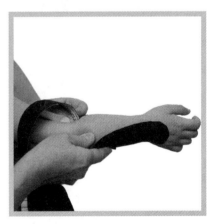

- Anchor the tape on the proximal third of the forearm (on volar surface)

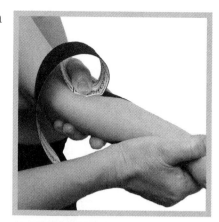

- Flex the elbow 20° - 45°
- Leave a space between the proximal and distal anchor
- Apply the distal anchor at the supraglenoid tubercle

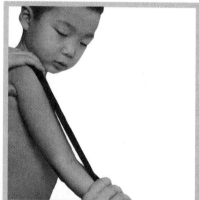

- Extend the elbow and gently rub down the tape over the biceps

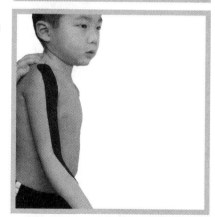

- Completed taping for postural alignment
- This technique can be used as an assist for elbow flexion and bringing hand to mouth

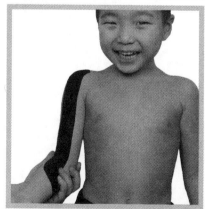

TRUNK

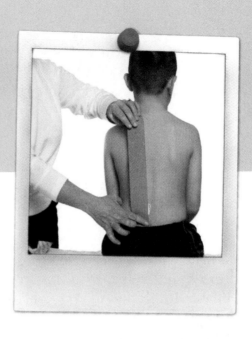

Abdominals

Rectus Abdominis
Origin: 5th, 6th, 7th, rib and xiphoid process of sternum
Insertion: pubic crest and symphysis
Action: flexion of the thorax and pelvis anteriorly, flexion of the trunk

Obliques External
Origin: 5th-12th rib
Insertion: linea alba, abdominal aponeurosis and iliac crest
Action: acting bilaterally, flexion of trunk; acting unilaterally, lateral flexion and rotation of trunk to opposite side

Obliques Internal
Origin: inguinal ligament, iliac crest, and thoracolumbar fascia
Insertion: 9th -12th rib, linea alba, with transverses abdominis into crest of pubis
Action: acting bilaterally, flexion of trunk; acting unilaterally, lateral flexion, rotation of the trunk to same side

Transverse Abdominis
Origin: 7th-12th rib, inguinal ligament, thoracolumbar fascia, iliac crest
Insertion: abdominal aponeurosis and linea alba, pubis
Action: acts like a girdle, compresses abdominal contents

Assessment of the abdominal muscles is important in the evaluation of trunk and pelvic alignment. In standing, the lateral fibers of the external and internal obliques act together assisting in maintaining the pelvis and thorax in proper postural alignment. Weakness in the abdominal musculature often presents as a greater anterior pelvic tilt, resulting in a lordotic standing posture. Abdominal weakness may also present as a more posterior pelvic tilt in sitting.

Based on the evaluation previously discussed (developmental milestones), the sequential development of postural control for the three planes of the body is sagittal first, frontal second and lastly, transverse. Children with asymmetrical posture and alignment require midline control and facilitation of symmetry. There must be control in the lateral and rotational planes for development of functional movement and positions.

A child with hypotonia may present with a wide base of support in sitting or standing, and a greater anterior pelvic tilt in standing with the center of gravity displaced forward. In bench sitting, the rectus abdominus may be tight or dominant, with an increase in posterior pelvic tilt; as the abdominal oblique muscles assist in bringing the trunk forward over the pelvis in sitting. Decreased abdominal muscle activity interferes with the development of righting and equilibrium responses. Kinesio® Taping to facilitate the internal and external abdominal obliques, combined with activities to activate the abdominal muscles in controlled movement, will assist in the development of balance and equilibrium reactions. These activities might include displacing the center of gravity in all directions for graded co-contraction of trunk flexors and extensors in functional activities.

The rectus abdominus is often a dominant muscle used in children with CNS dysfunction. The tendency for these children is to move in a straight plane of flexion and extension. There is poor rotational control and the rectus abdominus is dominant and short, pulling the sacrum and pelvis closer together with flaring of the 7th to 12th ribs laterally. Prior to any Kinesio® Taping techniques used to facilitate abdominals, it is essential to provide activities in prone or over a therapy ball in prone or supine to lengthen the rectus abdominus and also to mobilize the rib cage. Assess for range of motion in all trunk movement (flexion, extension, lateral flexion and rotation). Muscle length is necessary for trunk control and graded active movement.

Abdominal muscles help to stabilize the rib cage and work synergistically, interdigitating with the serratus anterior to stabilize the scapula and provide shoulder girdle stability. Weakness of the external and internal obliques may decrease respiratory capacity. In addition, muscle imbalance may present as shortening of musculature on one side of the trunk with over lengthening and stretch weakness on the opposite side.

The internal and external oblique muscles work synergistically to rotate the trunk. The transverses abdominis is the deepest of the abdominal muscles and wraps around the lower trunk like a girdle, to pull in the abdomen. Refined control of the trunk is not possible without muscle group interaction. Observe the child in all planes at rest and in transitions (i.e. prone, supine, sit).

In assessment, determine the primary cause of postural malalignment prior to the application of Kinesio® Tex tape. Ongoing evaluation is critical to ensure that the desired goals for alignment, function, and quality of movement are achieved through appropriate taping. Finally, dorsal trunk stabilizers (extensors and lower trapezius) may need to be taped in conjunction with abdominals to provide improved muscle balance.

- An angle finder can be used to measure the sacral angle of the child prior to taping the abdominal to assess change before and after the tape application (Cusick, 1997)

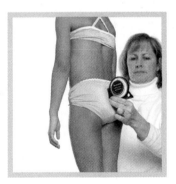

Internal and External Abdominal Obliques

Two 1.5 inch or 2inch "I" tapes
Recommendation: stretch rectus abdominus and thoracic spine and anterior spinal ligament, as well as mobilize ribcage prior to tape application.

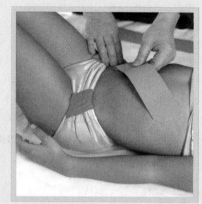

- Measure tape length from ASIS (anterior superior iliac spine) to the opposite lateral 10th rib

- Place the child supine, with hips flexed to place the pelvis in a more neutral position

- Anchor tape at the anterior superior iliac spine (ASIS) and apply toward umbilicus with paper-off tension

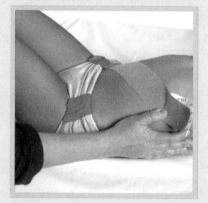

- Once reaching the umbilicus, have the child slightly side bend toward the same side where the anchor starts, to lengthen the opposite lateral trunk

- Apply the tape with paper-off tension diagonally over umbilicus toward lateral ribs 10 to 12, while using the other hand to bring the ribs down

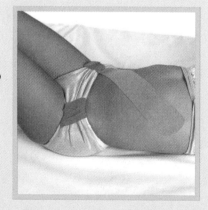

- End the tape on the ribs with no tension

- Bring the trunk back to midline position to apply tape to the opposite side

- Anchor the tape on the opposite anterior superior iliac spine and repeat the taping technique described previously

- Completed application will form an "X"

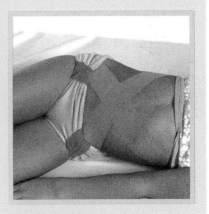

Transverse Abdominis:

This taping technique may be added to taping for abdominal oblique muscles

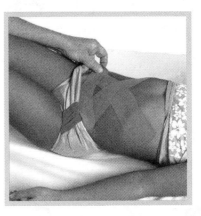

- Position the child in supine, with knees flexed
- If possible have the child perform a forceful exhalation (blow out)
- Kinesio® Tape is applied with paper-off tension across the lower abdomen, from ASIS to ASIS

Internal and External Obliques
Alternate method

Two 1.5 inch or 2 inch "Y" tapes

Purpose: this method stabilizes the ribs to "connect" upper and lower trunk and provide a more stable base for the shoulder girdle to move on. It can also be used if a gastrostomy tube is in place and needs to be considered in taping.

- Measure tape length from ASIS (anterior superior iliac spine) to the opposite lateral 10th rib
- Cut tape into "Y" with tails extending from umbilicus to ribs
- Place child supine, hips flexed to place pelvis in a more neutral position
- Anchor the tape at ASIS and apply diagonally over umbilicus with paper-off tension

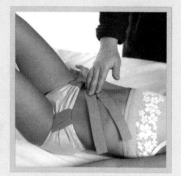

- Once reaching the umbilicus, where the split in the "Y" tape occurs, have the child slightly side bend to the opposite side to lengthen the lateral trunk
- Apply medial/superior tail toward anterior-lateral ribs 10 to 12 with minimal tension, while using the other hand to bring the ribs down toward the pelvis

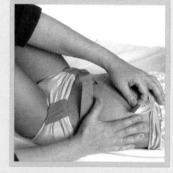

- With the child in the elongated position apply lateral/inferior tail towards the posterior-lateral ribs 10 to 12 with paper-off tension, again while bringing the ribs down

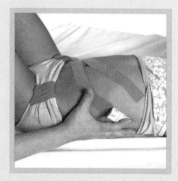

- When applying the second piece of Kinesio® Tape on the opposite side, be sure the child is back in midline position
- Anchor the tape on the opposite ASIS and repeat the taping procedure described previously

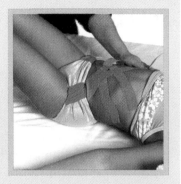

- Completed taping technique of the abdominals using "Y" taping
- May add transverse abdominis taping to this technique

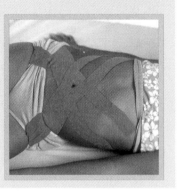

Split Lateral Trunk

Two 2 inch "X" tapes

This method may be used in conjunction with previous methods or individually. Tape is applied to lateral trunk to "connect" upper and lower trunk. Tension on tails can be adjusted to place more force in a specific area or on one side. One example for this application would be a child with hemiplegia who has range of motion to elongate the involved side, but tends to hold lateral trunk in a shortened position. Tape is applied to the uninvolved side to facilitate the elongation with weight shift on the more involved side.

- The child is placed side lying, with a roll under the mid-trunk to place the lateral trunk to be taped at a slight stretch
- The knees may be slightly flexed to keep pelvis in a more neutral position
- The center of "X" is anchored with no tension on the lateral trunk, midway between the iliac crest and the inferior ribcage

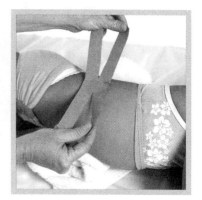

- The tails are applied with paper-off tension, unless different tension on each tail is indicated for alignment
- Anterior tails are applied to extend to pubis and toward inferior sternum
- *Note:* depending on the goal, the application of the taping technique may vary. The tape can be applied to the posterior tails initially versus anterior tails, and the tension on tails can be adjusted to place more force in a specific area or on one side

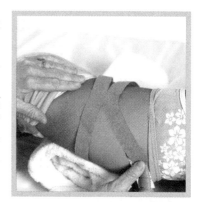

- Posterior tails are applied to extend to lower thoracic area and to pelvis
- Paper-off tension is used, unless otherwise determined by assessment

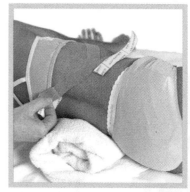

- Taping may be done unilaterally or bilaterally with more tension on one side
- This effect can also be achieved by removing the roll on the side during application, to create more tension on the tape

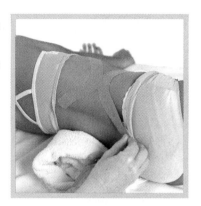

- Completed taping technique

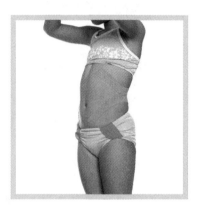

Trunk Extension

Erector Spinae

Origin: sacrum, iliac crest, lower thoracic vertebrae, transverse and spinous processes, and lower ribs

Insertion: transverse processes of C2 to the lumbar transverse processes

Action: extends and laterally flexes the trunk

Two 2 inch "I" tapes

- Measure tape length from sacrum to upper thoracic spine
- Tape may be applied with patient sitting. Try to avoid prone, as may be applied too tightly.
- May also use two 2" strips, placed on each side of the vertebral column, extending above and below weakest area
- This technique can be combined with abdominal taping for trunk stabilization

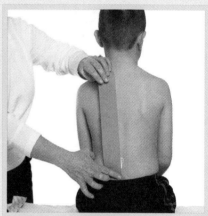

- Anchor the tape near sacrum, or if targeting an area, at least one level below
- Cue , or assist, the patient to hold an upright position
- Apply the tape, with paper-off tension, along the paraspinals
- Repeat on the opposite side
- Evaluate the tension required on each side of the spinous processes, and apply the tape with appropriate tension to facilitate midline posture. For example the right side may be more over lenghthen than the left.
- No tension is applied to the end of the tape

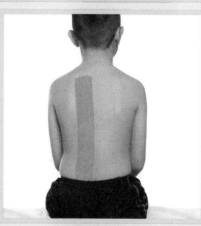

- Completed taping for trunk extension

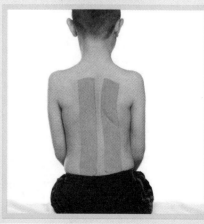

Alternate Technique 1:
Two 2 inch "Y" strips

- Measure tape length from sacrum to upper thoracic spine
- Tape may be applied with patient sitting. Try to avoid prone, as may be applied too tightly
- May also use two "Y" strips, placed on each side of the vertebral column
- This technique can be combined with abdominal taping for trunk stabilization

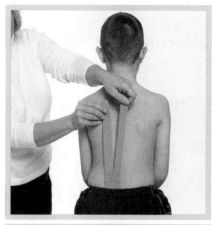

- Anchor the tape near sacrum, or if targeting an area, at least one level below
- Cue or assist the patient to hold an upright position
- Apply the medial tail, with paper-off tension, along the paraspinals
- No tension is applied to the end of the tape

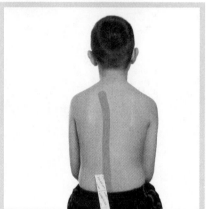

- Apply the lateral tail, with paper-off tension, along the paraspinals
- No tension is applied to the end of the tape

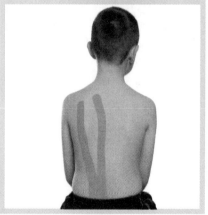

> **i** More tension may be applied to the lateral tail to facilitate trunk shortening on an over lengthened side. This may be indicated for the uninvolved side of a child with hemiplegia

- Completed taping for trunk extension

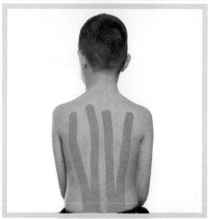

TRUNK

Alternate Technique 2:
Two 2 or 3 inch fan tapes

- Apply as previous "I" tapes
- Four tails on fan applied with paper-off tension

i This technique may provide more sensory input to extensors over a wider area

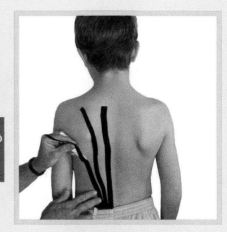

- Fan taping to facilitate trunk extension
- This technique is usually done bilaterally

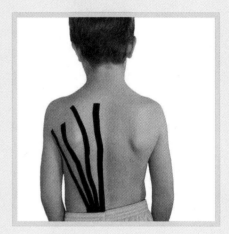

Latissimus Dorsi

Origin: T7-L5, posterior sacrum and posterior iliac crest via the thoracolumbar fascia
Insertion: Intertubercular groove of the humerus
Action: Medially rotates, adducts, extends arm at the shoulder joint. With the arm fixed the
            latissimus dorsi anteriorly tilts and clerates the pelvis at the lumbosacral joint.

Latissimus Dorsi Assist

The latissimus dorsi elevates the pelvis and trunk toward the arm, which is crucial for a child who is required to perform pressure relief while seated in a wheelchair, to use crutches for walking, or to transfer in and out of a wheelchair. Kinesio® Taping the latissimus dorsi may provide assist to the lower back during these activities, which require the use of upper body strength.

A 1.5 or 2 inch "I" tape

- Ask the patient to sit or stand "tall" or straight
- Measure the tape from the posterior superior iliac spine (PSIS) to the posterior aspect of the axillary area
- Anchor the tape at the PSIS

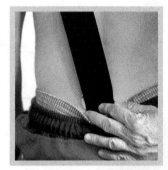

- Hold the arm in shoulder internal rotation (turned in)
- Apply the tape with paper-off tension toward the insertion of the latissimus dorsi, on the posterior and medial humerus by the axillary region
- No tension is applied at the end of the tape

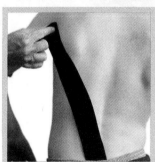

- Completed taping to assist the latissimus dorsi

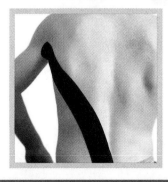

Alternate Taping for Latissimus Dorsi Elongation

Tightness or shortening of the trunk laterally can occur because of limited passive and active range of motion of the latissimus dorsi. Length of the muscle must be provided through a positioning and stretching program. Active reach can be limited due to the resistance of the latissimus dorsi. Applying Kinesio® Tape from insertion to origin with the latissimus dorsi in an elongated position will assist with decreasing the tightness and assist with improving active arm movement needed for function.

A 1.5 or 2 inch "I" tape

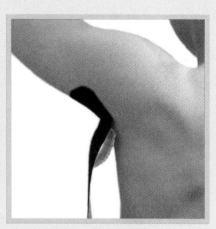

- Measure the "I" tape from the axillary region on the posterior medial side of the humerus, down the rib cage diagonally toward the PSIS
- Position arm in humeral flexion and external rotation, above shoulder level, as the trunk is elongated on the same side. This puts the latissimus dorsi in a fully lengthened position.
- Anchor the tape on the posterior medial aspect of the humerus

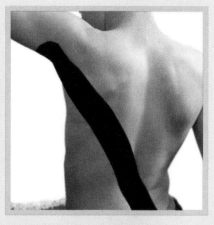

- Apply tape with paper-off tension, diagonally toward the posterior superior iliac spine (PSIS)
- Technique may be done with trunk flexed. If the trunk is not flexed, more stability is provided to the lumbar area

- Completed taping

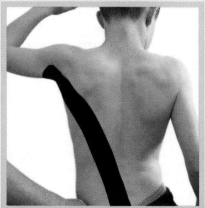

Disc Herniation / Protrusion

Six 2 inch "I" tape, a 2 inch "Y" tape

- Tear the tape backing in the center and fold back the edges on all six pieces of tape
- Have the patient lean forward over a table into trunk flexion, with a posterior pelvic tilt
- Take 50-75% of the tension out from the center of the first piece of tape, and with downward pressure, apply the tape in a horizontal plane
- No tension is applied at the end of the tape

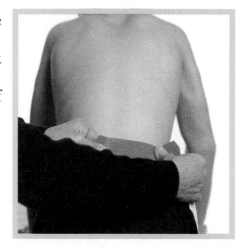

- Repeat the procedure
- Take 50-75% of the tension out from the center of the second piece of tape, and with downward pressure, apply the tape in a vertical plane
- No tension is applied at the end of the tape

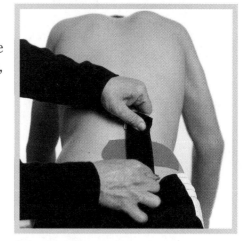

- Repeat the procedure with the third, diagonal piece
- Take 50-75% of the tension out from the center of the third and fourth piece of tape, and with downward pressure, apply the tape in a diagonal plane
- No tension is applied at the end of the tape

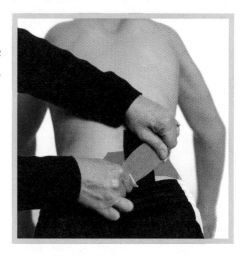

- Repeat the procedure with the fourth, diagonal piece
- Take 50-75% of the tension out from the center of the third and fourth piece of tape, and with downward pressure, apply the tape in a diagonal plane
- No tension is applied at the end of the tape
- The end taping looks like a star or flower and is often referred to as the "disc star"

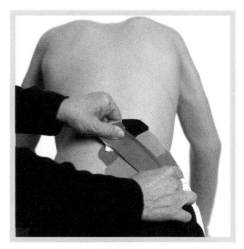

- A "Y" tape is then applied, with paper-off tension, anchoring at the sacrum
- The child maintains the posterior tilt and trunk flexion (as tolerated) as the tails are applied
- Tails are applied with paper-off tension, one on each side of the spine, to support the paraspinals
- Two "I" tapes could also be used

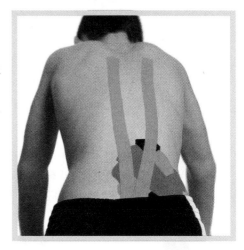

LOWER EXTREMITY

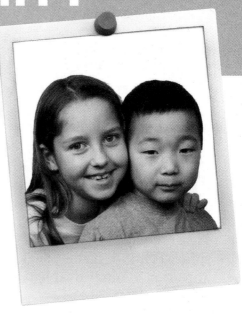

Tight Iliotibial Band

Tensor Fascia Lata
Origin: anterior iliac crest
Insertion: into iliotibial band to lateral tibial condyle
Action: flexes, medial rotates and abducts the hip joint, tenses fascia lata, and assists in knee extension

The iliotibial band is a wide, thick band of fascia, with numerous attachments to the entire leg, extending from the pelvis to below the knee. Restriction of this band can cause "clicking" and pain at the hip or greater trochanter, as well as knee pain. The iliotibial band often becomes dominant or tight in children with CNS involvement, who move in a flexion pattern. Tightness is also observed in children with low muscle tone and decreased proximal stability, as they use a wide base of support for balance. Adolescent athletes often have muscle imbalances of the lower extremity, and IT band tightness is prevalent.

A 2 or 3 inch "I" tape, or 2 overlapping 2 inch "I" tapes

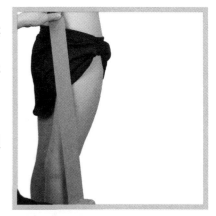

- Measure tape length from the posterior superior iliac spine (PSIS) to distal knee
- Tape can be applied in sidelying, on opposite side, or in standing

Standing technique:
- Position the child in upright posture with the hip adducted and extended
- Anchor the tape lateral to PSIS

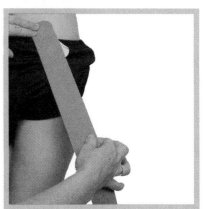

- Instruct the child to laterally flex the trunk toward opposite side
- Apply the tape with paper-off tension, diagonally to lateral hip and over the greater trochanter

- Apply the tape, with paper-off tension, down lateral thigh over IT band

ℹ Remember the iliotibial band often becomes displaced anteriorly as it becomes restricted

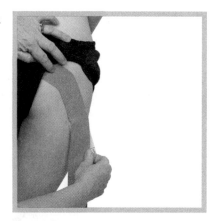

- Apply tape, with paper-off tension, Continue taping down lateral thigh over IT band, ending distal to the knee

ℹ If pain is present at the lateral knee, tape may be applied by anchoring at the knee and applying with paper-off tension to the PSIS

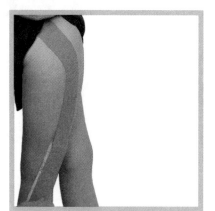

- Completed taping, in standing, for iliotibial band tightness

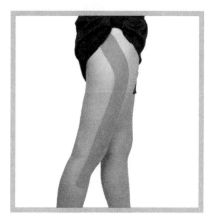

Sidelying technique:
- Anchor tape with the leg abducted, and then adduct the leg with neutral extension and rotation
- Anchor the tape at the posterior iliac crest
- Apply the tape with paper-off tension, diagonally to lateral hip and over the greater trochanter

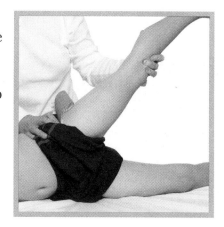

- Apply tape with paper-off tension, down lateral thigh over IT band to end on the thigh or distal to the knee

ℹ Remember the iliotibial band often becomes displaced anteriorly as it becomes restricted

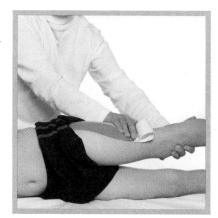

- Completed taping, in sidelying, for iliotibial band tightness

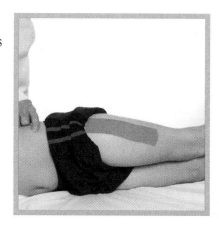

Piriformis Relaxation

This technique targets the piriformis muscle, as well as the other deep hip lateral rotators. The piriformis is the most superior of the deep lateral rotators. It is difficult to palpate, but can be palpated between the posterior superior iliac spine (PSIS), between the border of the sacrum and the greater trochanter, during active hip lateral rotation.

The sciatic nerve lies between the deep lateral rotators of the femur and the piriformis.

Origin: Anterior sacrum and sacral ligament
Insertion: Greater trochanter
Action: Lateral rotation of the femur

A 2 inch "Y" strip

- Measure the tape from the greater trochanter over the gluteal area toward the sacroiliac joint

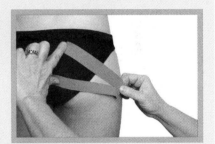

- Position the hip in medial rotation and flexion and anchor the tape at the greater trochanter
- Apply the superior tail with paper-off tension along the superior gluteal area toward the sacroiliac joint

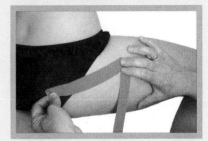

- Apply the inferior tail with paper-off tension along the inferior gluteal area toward the sacroiliac joint

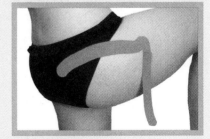

- Completed taping for piriformis relaxation

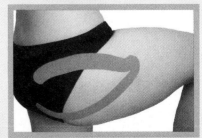

ℹ This technique is often done with IT band space correction taping. The IT band migrates anteriorly as it shortens, which may place increased tension on the piriformis, presenting as SI pain or gluteal tenderness.

Groin Pull

Hip Adductors
Origin: from pubis to ischium
Insertion: length of medial border of femur
Action: adduct the leg and slight outward rotation

A 2 or 3 inch "I" tape

- Measure the tape length from the groin to the distal knee
- Place the child in supine with the knee flexed 90° and the hip adducted to neutral and flexed to about 45°
- Anchor tape just distal to groin medially

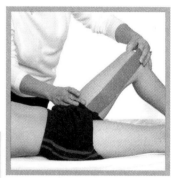

i A 3 inch wide piece of tape may be used if child is larger, or more support is needed

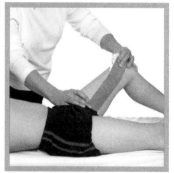

- Apply the tape with paper-off tension, as the leg is abducted and the hip and knee are slowly extended

- End the tape just distal to the medial knee
- No tension is applied at the end of the tape
- A corrective piece of tape, with full tension taken from the center, may be applied perpendicular to this piece over the area of pain

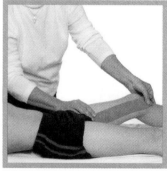

- Completed taping for a groin pull or adductor strain

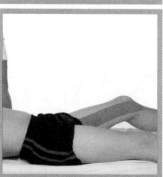

Hip Abduction / Extension

The technique to facilitate hip abduction is similar to the taping technique to facilitate hip lateral rotation, but the focus of taping is on the hip abduction, more than the rotation. This technique will also provide support for single leg stance activities and for the stance phase of gait.

Gluteus Maximus
Origin: medial iliac crest, sacrum, coccyx, and sacrotuberous ligament
Insertion: proximal part- iliotibial band, distal part-gluteal tuberosity of femur
Action: extends, laterally rotates the hip,
             Lower fibers assist in adduction of the hip joint and upper fibers assist in abduction.
             Through insertion into iliotibial tract, it helps stabilize knee in extension

Gluteus Medius
Origin: upper posterior surface of ilium
Insertion: great trochanter of femur
Action: abduction of the hip joint. Anterior fibers medially rotate hip and may assist hip
             flexion, posterior fiber laterally rotate hip and assist hip extension.

One or two 2 inch "I" tapes

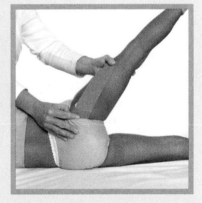

- Measure tape length from sacrum, diagonal over lateral thigh, to above the knee
- Position the child sidelying, in a relaxed position
- For optimal alignment, hip should be extended to neutral, abducted 40° to 45°, and slightly laterally rotated
- A second person may need to hold the hip into lateral rotation, with the knee extended

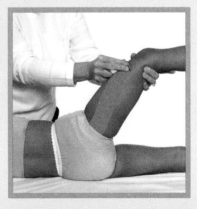

- Anchor the tape on the sacral area with no tension
- Apply the tape with paper-off tension, wrapping the tape diagonally around the greater trochanter to lateral mid thigh

- Completed taping to facilitate hip abduction
- A second piece of tape, overlapping the first, may be applied for increased support
- Observe the position of the lower extremity after taping, in sitting, standing and gait, if able

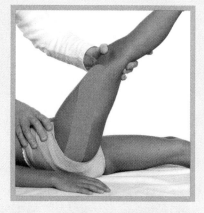

- Measure tape length from sacrum, diagonal over lateral thigh, to above the knee
- Position the child in standing
- For optimal alignment, hip should be extended to neutral, abducted 40° to 45°, and slightly laterally rotated

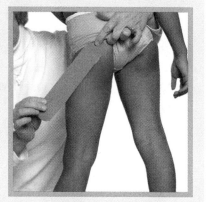

- Ask child to hold their hand on their hip, with the hip stabilized forward
- Gently rotate the hip laterally
- A second person may need to hold the hip into lateral rotation, with the knee extended
- Anchor the tape on the sacral area with no tension

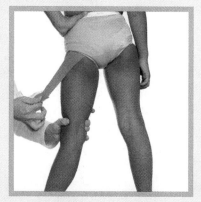

- Apply the tape with paper-off tension, wrapping the tape diagonally around the greater trochanter to lateral mid-thigh
- No tension is applied at the end of the tape

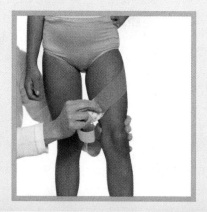

Kinesio Taping® in Pediatrics

LOWER EXTREMITY

- Completed taping to facilitate hip abduction
- A second piece of tape, overlapping the first, may be applied for increased support
- Observe the position of the lower extremity after taping, in sitting, standing and gait, if able

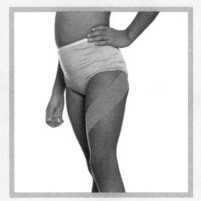

Hip Extension

To facilitate hip extension, Kinesio® Tape can be applied as previous, but with the hip positioned in slight abduction and more extension.

- Measure tape length from sacrum, diagonally toward postero-lateral thigh
- Position the patient standing
- For optimal alignment, hip should be extended past neutral, abducted 40 to 45°, and slightly laterally rotated

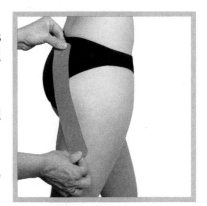

- Anchor the tape on the sacral area with no tension
- Apply the tape with paper-off tension, wrapping the tape diagonally toward the postero-lateral mid-thigh

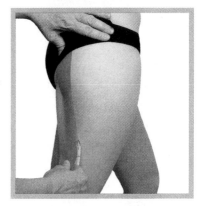

- Completed taping for hip extension

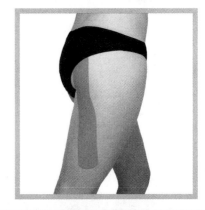

Hip Lateral Rotation

Gluteus Maximus

Origin: medial iliac crest, sacrum, coccyx, and sacrotuberous ligament
Insertion: proximal part- iliotibial band, distal part-gluteal tuberosity of femur
Action: extends, laterally rotates the hip,
            Lower fibers assist in adduction of the hip joint and upper fibers assist in abduction.
            Through insertion into iliotibial tract, it helps stabilize knee in extension

Gluteus Medius

Origin: upper posterior surface of ilium
Insertion: great trochanter of femur
Action: abduction of the hip joint. Anterior fibers medially rotate hip and may assist hip
            flexion, posterior fiber laterally rotate hip and assist hip extension.

Full-term newborn babies have about forty degrees of medial femoral torsion, which decreases with boney modeling throughout childhood and adolescence. Knowledge of the normal range of motion for specific ages is essential for taping.

In evaluating lower extremity rotational issues the following must be considered:
(See Cusick, 1997)
- Evaluate pelvic alignment
- Assess hip medial and lateral rotation
- Assess femoral torsion with the Ryders Test (Cusick 1997)
- Assess thigh/foot angle
- Assess tibio-fibular rotation
- Assess transmalleolar axis
- Assess for available range of motion, mobility and alignment.

Know how much lateral rotation is available at the hip, assessing hip medial and lateral rotation, as well as Ryder's test for medial femoral torsion in prone. Excess force into lateral rotation when range is limited, will cause injurious torque forces on the head of the femur and the hip capsule. If lateral rotation is available, but excessive medial rotation is present, taping can limit amount of medial rotation available.
NEVER FORCE LATERAL ROTATION AT THE HIP WHEN MEDIAL FEMORAL TORSION IS INCREASED and bony alignment is the primary problem.

Mobilization and myofascial release techniques to improve mobility, may be required prior to taping. Determine the goal position to be achieved and assess results after tape is applied.
This technique may be done in standing or sidelying, though sidelying should be considered initially for consistency in application.

One or two 2 inch "I" tapes

- Measure tape length from sacrum, diagonal over lateral thigh, to above the knee
- Position the patient sidelying, in a relaxed position
- For optimal alignment, hip should be extended to neutral, abducted 20° to 30°, and laterally rotated
- A second person may need to hold the hip into lateral rotation, with the knee extended

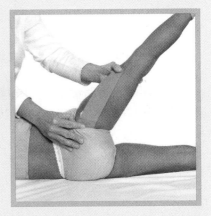

- Anchor the tape on the sacral area with no tension
- Apply the tape with paper-off tension, wrapping the tape diagonally around the greater trochanter to lateral mid-thigh

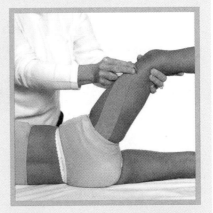

- Completed taping to facilitate hip lateral rotation
- A second piece of tape, overlapping the first, may be applied for increased support
- Observe the position of the lower extremity after taping, both in standing and gait, if able

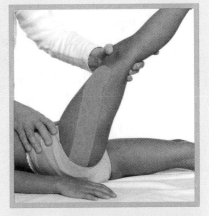

- Measure tape length from sacrum, diagonal over lateral thigh, to above the knee
- Position the child in standing
- For optimal alignment, hip should be extended to neutral, abducted 20° to 30°, and laterally rotated

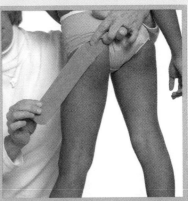

- Ask the child to hold their hand on their hip, with the hip stabilized forward
- Gently rotate the hip laterally
- A second person may need to hold the hip into lateral rotation, with the knee extended
- Anchor the tape on the sacral area with no tension

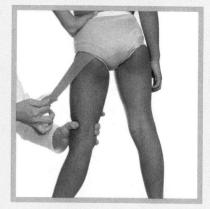

- Apply the tape with paper-off tension, wrapping the tape diagonally around the greater trochanter to lateral mid-thigh
- No tension is applied at the end of the tape

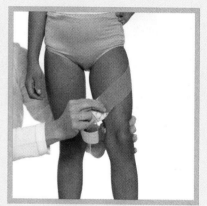

- Completed taping to facilitate hip lateral rotation
- A second piece of tape, overlapping the first, may be applied for increased support
- Observe the position of the lower extremity after taping, both in standing and gait, if able

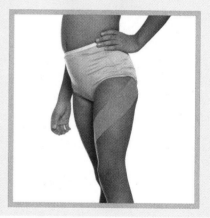

Hip Medial Rotation

Full-term newborn babies have about forty degrees of medial femoral torsion, which decreases with boney modeling throughout childhood and adolescence. Facilitation of increased medial rotation should be considered seriously before taping. Prior to taping for medial rotation of the hip, be sure femoral head is stable in the acetabulum.

Children may stand with a wide base of support, with hips in abduction and lateral rotation to increase stability. Taping may improve alignment, but needs to be accompanied by strengthening activities in weightbearing.

In evaluating lower extremity rotational issues the following must be considered:
(See Cusick, 1997)
- Evaluate pelvic alignment
- Assess hip medial and lateral rotation
- Assess femoral torsion with the Ryders Test (Cusick 1997)
- Assess thigh/foot angle
- Assess tibio-fibular rotation
- Assess transmalleolar axis
- Assess for available range of motion, mobility and alignment.

Mobilization and myofascial release techniques to improve mobility, may be required prior to taping. Determine the goal position to be achieved and assess results after tape is applied.
This technique may be done in standing or sidelying, though sidelying should be considered initially for consistency in application.

One or two 2 inch "I" tapes

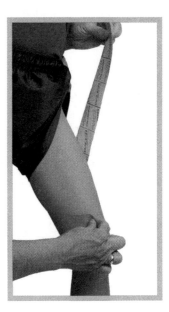

- Measure tape length proximal and superior to the medial knee, extending diagonally over posterior thigh, above lateral hip
- Position the child in standing or sidelying
- For optimal alignment, hip should be extended to neutral, abducted 10° to 20°, and medially rotated with minimal force
- A second person may need to hold the hip into medial rotation, with the knee extended

- Anchor the tape at the medial knee joint area with no tension
- Apply the tape with paper-off tension, wrapping the tape diagonally around the posterior knee and thigh

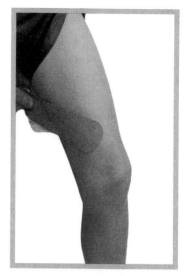

- Extend tape, with paper-off tension, above the lateral hip joint
- Completed taping to facilitate hip medial rotation
- No tension is applied at the end of the tape
- Tape should not extend over posterior gluteal folds, as it will limit hip flexion for sitting
- A second piece of tape, overlapping the first, may be applied for increased support

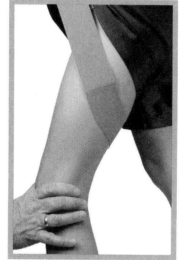
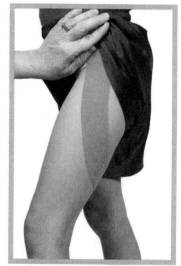

- Completed taping
- Observe the position of the lower extremity after taping, both in standing and gait, if able

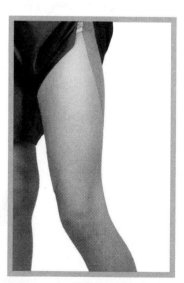

Quadriceps Assist

Quadriceps femoris
Origin: Dorsal section, external surface of ilium between iliac crest and posterior gluteal line, the central section, anterior gluteal line.
Gluteal aponeurosis.
Insertion: Oblique ridge of lateral surface of greater trochanter of femur.
Action: extends the knee

A 2 inch "Y" strip

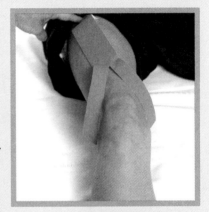

- Measure the tape length from the proximal thigh to the distal knee
- Tape "Y" is split at the musculotendinous junction of the quadruceps, above the patella
- Anchor the tape just distal to groin, on anterior surface of thigh
- Apply the tape with paper-off tension, along the belly of the quadriceps muscles

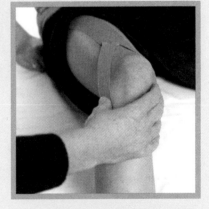

- Flex the knee an appropriate amount, determined by the amount of assistance required and the goal of the taping technique
- For assist with sit to stand, or end range of knee extension, minimal knee flexion is indicated

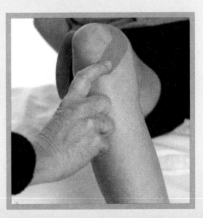

- Apply the medial tail with paper-off tension
- Tension may be placed near the end of the tails under the patella, if patellar tendonitis is present
- No tension is applied at the end of the tail

- Apply the lateral tail with paper-off tension
- More tension may be applied on medial or lateral tail to assist in alignment of the patella
- No tension is applied at the end of the tail

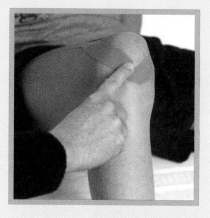

- Completed taping for quadruceps assist

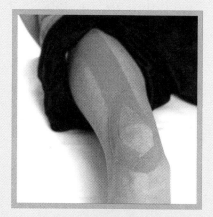

- May add taping for patellar tendonitis to quadriceps assist for additional proprioceptive input and support

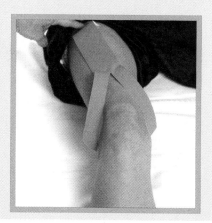

LOWER EXTREMITY

Knee Stabilization

This technique (insertion to origin) may be used for an acute quadriceps strain and also with the previous quad assist to provide support to the knee joint.

A 2 or 3 inch "Y" tape

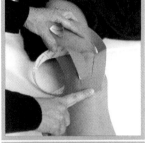

- Measure the tape length from the distal knee to the proximal thigh
- Flex the knee an appropriate amount, determined by the amount of assistance required and the goal of the taping technique
- For assist with sit to stand, or end range of knee extension, minimal knee flexion is indicated

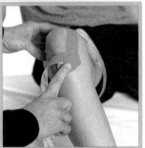

- Anchor the tape just distal to the knee joint, at the tibial tuberosity
- Apply the tape with paper-off tension, surrounding the patella and over the quadriceps muscles

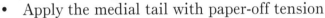

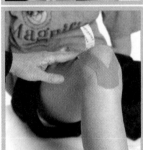

- Apply the medial tail with paper-off tension
- Apply the lateral tail with paper-off tension
- No tension is applied at the end of the tails

- Completed taping for knee stabilization

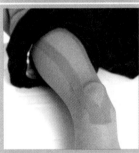

- May combine with quadriceps facilitation technique if indicated
- Can use taping techniques for quadriceps assist and modify to facilitate appropriate patellar tracking
- This can be done by placing more tension on the medial or lateral tails of the quadriceps taping

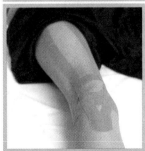

Patellar Tendonitis

Patellar tendonitis is often seen in adolescent athletes. Children go through rapid growth spurts, often creating additional muscle imbalances. The femur is the longest bone in the body, and as it grows, the range of motion in the quadriceps and hamstrings often becomes limited. A full lower extremity biomechanical assessment is essential to establish the cause of knee pain, and to assist in determining exercises to combine with the taping techniques chosen.

This technique can be used for adolescents with Osgood-Schlatters tibial tuberosity apophysitis.

A 2 inch "I" tape
Mechanical Assist

- Measure tape length as two times the length of the thigh
- Place the patient in supine, with the knee extended, or in standing
- Tear the tape backing at the center and fold back the edges
- Pull full tension from the center of the tape, as it is applied between the distal patella and the tibial tuberosity

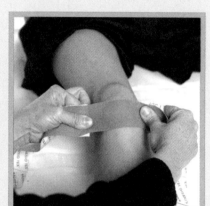

- Flex the knee 45° and apply the tape, with moderate tension, medial and lateral to patella
- Use the heel of your hand along the tape, to direct the tape

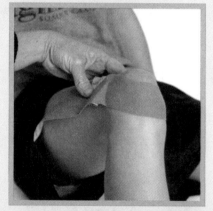

- Flex the knee 90° and apply the tape, with paper off tension, along medial and lateral border of quadriceps to proximal thigh
- No tension is applied at the end of the tape

ℹ This technique may be combined with a quadriceps assist, to give increased stability to the knee joint

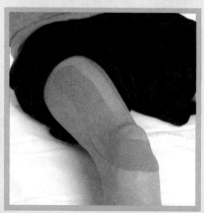

Patellar Alignment

Two 2 inch "Y" tapes
Mechanical Correction

- Place knee in 15° to 20° flexion, with knee over a bolster
- Start "Y" tapes at posterior aspect of the knee and apply tails over proximal and distal to patella with moderate tension
- Leave popliteal fossa open
- May only need to apply on medial side for lateral patellar tracking

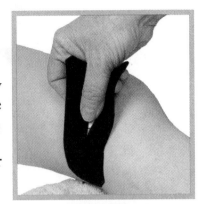

- An assessment of patellar tracking should be done, in closed chain if possible
- Apply tension to medial or lateral tails, depending on how patella tracks, as they come over the edges of the patella. Patella most often tracks laterally
- Tails will assist in guiding patella medially or laterally

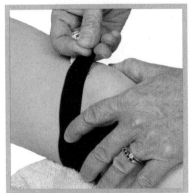

- No tension is applied at the end of the tails

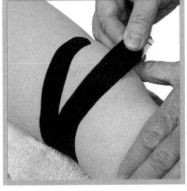

- Apply "Y" strips medial and lateral
- Apply to medial side first, if patella tracks laterally
- Remember, the patella tracks in the patellar groove

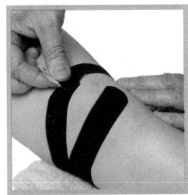

- Completed taping for patellar alignment
- Remember, tape will only be effective if patella requires minimal assist to correct

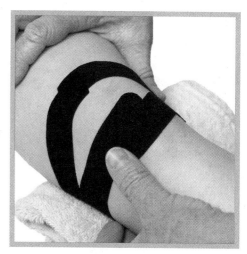

- If patella tracks laterally may combine application of medial Y tape with a mechanical assist along the lateral surface of the patella

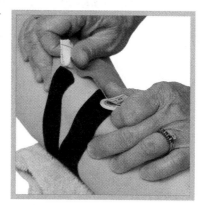
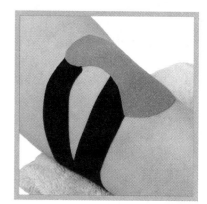

- May combine with quadriceps facilitation technique if indicated
- Can use taping techniques for quadriceps assist and modify to facilitate appropriate patellar tracking
- This can be done by placing more tension on the medial or lateral tails of the quadriceps taping,
- Assess position at rest and with movement

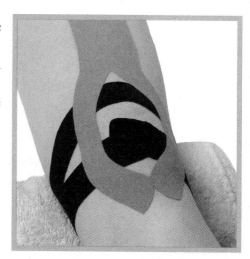

Patella Alta: Mechanical Correction

Patella alta is often seen in children and adults with CNS involvement. The patella needs to be mobilized prior to taping. Patellar alignment is key to the optimal force of the quadriceps for knee extension. This taping is often combined with a quadriceps taping technique.

Three 2 inch "I" tapes
Mechanical Correction

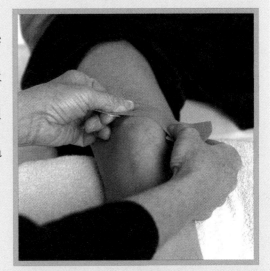

- Tape length is 3 to 4 inches
- Child is positioned in supine or sitting, with knee supported and flexed 15°
- Tear the tape backing at the center and fold back the edges of all three pieces of tape
- Apply the first piece of tape diagonally on medial knee joint, overlapping the patella by half
- Use minimal force on thumbs to position patella downward
- Tape is applied with paper-off tension
- No tension is applied at the end of the tape

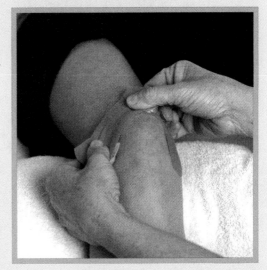

- Apply the second piece of tape diagonally on the lateral knee joint, overlapping the patella by half
- Use minimal force on thumbs to position patella downward and medial
- Tape is applied with paper-off tension
- No tension is applied at the end of the tape

- Apply the third piece of tape superiorly on the knee joint, overlapping the patella by half
- Use minimal force on thumbs to position patella further downward
- Tape is applied with paper-off tension
- No tension is applied at the end of the tape

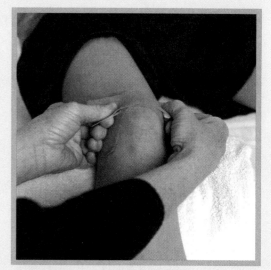

- Completed taping for patella alta

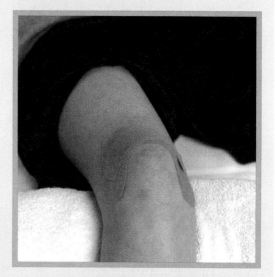

- Taping to bring patella toward joint line, when patella alta is present, may be combined with quadruceps facilitation technique

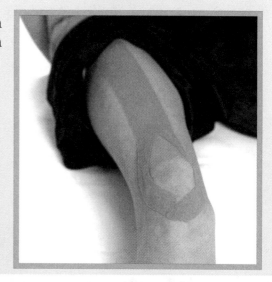

Hamstring Taping

Hamstrings
Origin: Biceps femoris: Long head: ischial tuberosity, short head on upper femur
               Semimembranosis/ semitendonosis: ischial tuberosity
Insertion: Biceps femoris: lateral tibial condyle and lateral head of the fibula
               Semimembranosis/ semitendonosis: medial tibial condyle (peps anserine)
Action: Biceps femoris: flexes knee and outwardly rotates knee when flexed, extends hip
               Semimembranosis/ semitendonosis: flexes knee and inwardly rotates knee when
               flexed, extends hip

Technique 1: Hamstring Pull
A 2 inch "Y" tape, a 2 inch "I" tape

- Measure tape length from ischial tuberosity to the knee joint
- The tails of the "Y" tape are two-thirds of the tape length
- Place the child in a prone position, with the knee extended
- Anchor the tape just distal to the gluteal fold below the ischial tuberosity, on the posterior thigh

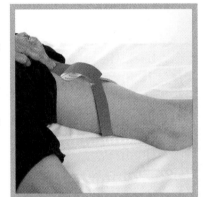

- Flex the knee and have the child extend the knee as the medial tail is applied, with paper-off tension, to posterio-medial knee

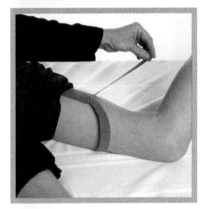

Flex the knee and have the child extend the knee as the lateral tail is applied, with paper-off tension, to posterio-lateral knee

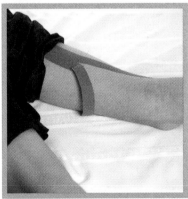

- This technique can also be done in standing, or with a 3 inch wide tape on an adult

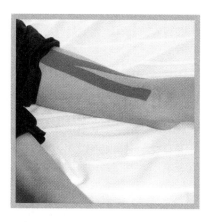

- A corrective strip may be applied over the pulled or painful area
- Tear the backing from the center of the "I" tape and fold back the edges
- Take full tension from center of the corrective strip and apply perpendicular to the previous tape, directly over the painful area
- A second corrective tape may be added, overlapping the first

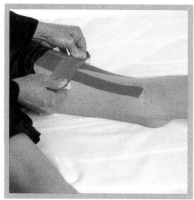

- Completed taping for a hamstring pull

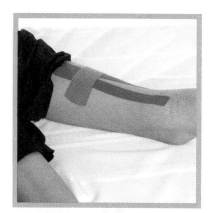

Technique 2: Hamstring relaxation
Kinesio® Tex tape can be applied on the hamstring, from insertion to origin in a fully lengthened position, using two 1 or 2 inch "I" tapes.

Two 2 inch "I" tapes

- It is helpful, but not necessary to measure hamstring length before and after taping to assess changes. One method used is the hamstring length test using the popliteal angle (Cusick 1997)
- Initial and maximal end-range should be recorded

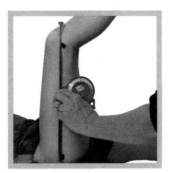
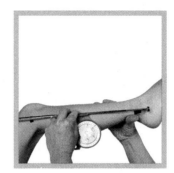

- Measure tape from distal knee when extended to ischial tuberosity with hip flexed
- Position the leg in knee extension and anchor the tape to the lateral inferior knee, at the hamstring insertion
- The first tape is applied with paper-off tension and the knee extended, from the lateral hamstring tendon to the midthigh

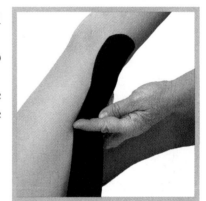

- The knee and hip are then flexed

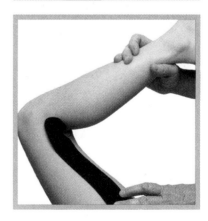

- The hip is the flexed fully, and the tape application continues with paper-off tension, to the ischial tuberosity

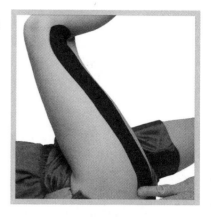

- The second tape is applied from the distal medial hamstring tendon to the ischial tuberosity, in the same manner

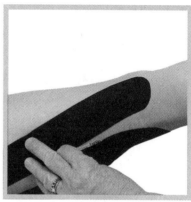

- Completed taping for a hamstring relaxation

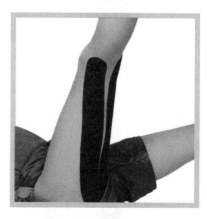

Knee Lateral Rotation

Assessment of the thigh-foot angle and tibio-fibular rotation should be done prior to taping. (Cusick, 1997). Knowledge of normal range of motion for specific ages is essential.

One or two 2 inch "I" tapes

- Measure tape length from the middle of the lower leg, diagonally behind the knee, to the midthigh
- A second person may be needed to stabilize the upper thigh and rotate the lower leg medially, with minimal force
- Anchor tape on lower leg, directed laterally, at a diagonal to pass over the popliteal crease

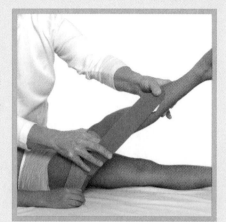

- Apply the tape, with paper-off tension, diagonally over the popliteal space, to upper thigh

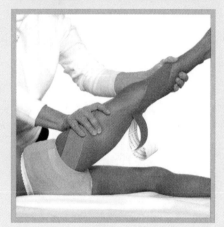

- Tape ends at the anterior midthigh
- No tension is applied at the end of the tape

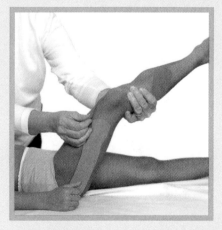

- Completed taping to facilitate knee lateral rotation
- Prior to and after taping, asses the lower extremity position in standing and the forward progression angle of gait

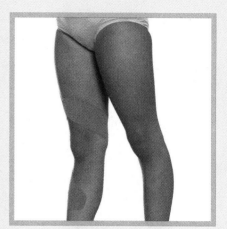

- This technique is often combined with taping to facilitate hip lateral rotation

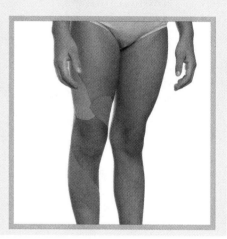

Knee Medial Rotation

Assessment of the thigh-foot angle and tibio-fibular rotation should be done prior to taping. (Cusick, 1997). Knowledge of normal range of motion for specific ages is essential.

One or two 2 inch "I" tapes

- Measure tape length from the middle of the lower leg, diagonally behind the knee, to the midthigh
- A second person may be needed to stabilize the upper thigh and rotate the lower leg medially, with minimal force
- Anchor tape on lower leg, directed medially, at a diagonal to pass over the popliteal crease

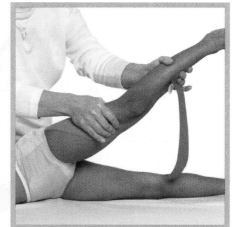

- Apply the tape, with paper-off tension, diagonally over the popliteal space, to upper thigh

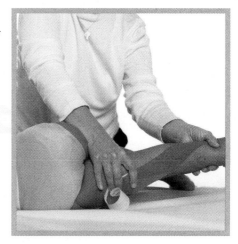

- Tape ends at the anterior midthigh
- No tension is applied at the end of the tape

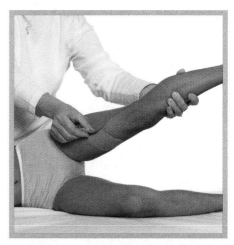

- Completed taping to facilitate knee medial rotation
- Prior to and after taping, assess the lower extremity position in standing and the forward progression angle of gait

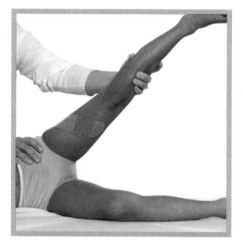

- Anterior view of taping to facilitate knee medial rotation

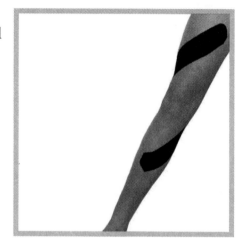

- Posterior view of taping to facilitate knee medial rotation

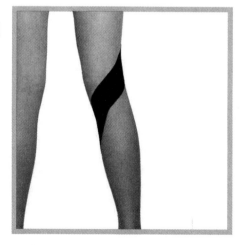

Knee Hyperextension

Prior to taping for knee hyperextension, or recurvatum, assess mobility and alignment in the lower extremity. It is essential that function is not compromised with taping. If a child requires knee hyperextension to maintain standing, as in children with spinal muscular atrophy, muscular dystrophy or severe weakness, taping may not be appropriate Standing balance and control may be assesses during a therapy session, and time in the tape may be increased as endurance increases.

The primary cause of the knee hyperextension needs to be determined. Causative factors include: tight ankle plantarflexors, weak quadriceps, weak hamstrings, tight rectus femoris, and knee joint hypermobility. Prior to taping, determine the goal position to be achieved. For example, a goal of only 5 degrees of hyperextension, instead of 20 degrees hyperextension.

Two 2 inch "I" tapes
Functional Correction

- Document the femoro-fibular angle (also called standing knee angle) on the lateral leg, in relaxed stance (Cusick 1997)
- In looking at knee alignment, note if genu varum or valgum is present
- Assess strength to make sure quadriceps and hamstrings can stabilize knee when it is not in a hyperextended position
- Knee hyperextension may be mechanism used to gain stability in weightbearing when these muscles are weak

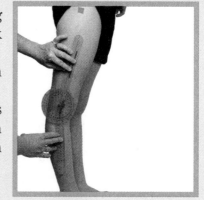

- Position the child in prone
- Support lower leg on towels or with second person to assist
- Tear the tape backing in the center and fold back the edges
- Place the first piece of tape diagonally in popliteal space, with no tension

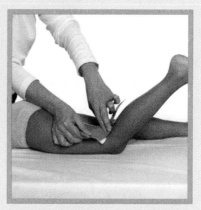

- Place the knee in about 30° to 45° of flexion
- Apply the two ends of the tape, with paper-off tension, diagonally toward anterior thigh and anterior lower leg
- No tension is applied on the last inch of tape

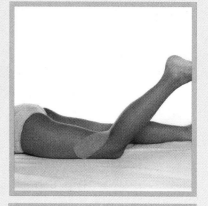

- Place the second piece of tape diagonally in popliteal space, with no tension
- This piece forms an "X" with the first piece
- Place the knee in about 30° to 45° of flexion
- Apply the two ends of the tape, with paper-off tension, diagonally toward anterior thigh and anterior lower leg
- No tension on the last inch of tape

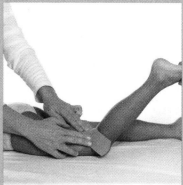

- Completed taping for knee hyperextension

The tension on the tape and force of the positioning assist, is determined by the amount of flexion the knee is placed in during the application.

If muscle tone and stiffness are dominant into LE extension, taping the knee alone may cause excess pressure on tissues and cause bruising.

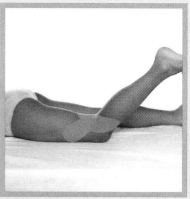

- A second set of tape may be added, overlapping first by one-half

- Evaluate alignment after taping to assure proper technique

- Have the child stand, and if appropriate ambulate with tape. The tape will loosen after a few steps. Tape can be added over tape, with knee in more flexion, if more flexion at the knee is indicated

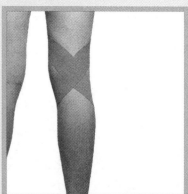

Be sure to take into consideration the fact that the knee joint may have been in a congruent position in hyperextension and the joint surfaces may have modeled to allow for this hyperextension.

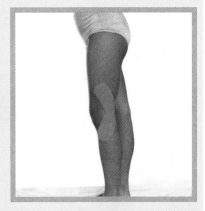

Placing the knee in a more neutral position may affect congruity of the joint and ligament stability, particularly in the anterior and posterior cruciates need to be assessed.

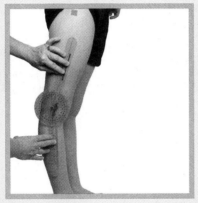

Knee position prior to taping

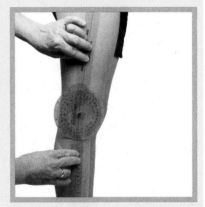

Knee position after taping

This technique may also be used to limit elbow hyperextension, though laxity in the ulnar collateral ligament must also be assessed.

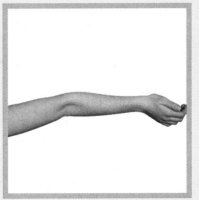

Elbow position prior to taping

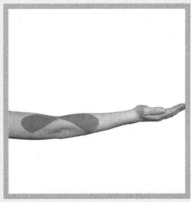

Elbow position after taping

Medial Tibial Stress Syndrome

Tibialis Posterior
Origin: interosseus membrane and adjacent surfaces of the tibia and fibula
Insertion: plantar side of tarsals, 2ⁿᵈ-4ᵗʰ metatarsals and calcaneus
Action: plantarflexes and inverts the ankle

Shin splints may be seen with inflammation of the tibialis posterior, tibialis anterior, or peronei muscle of the lower leg. A stress fracture must be ruled out. Taping is done insertion to origin to the affected muscle group to aid in a fascial release. Localized areas of pain are usually evident along the tibial crest. These painful "hot spots" may be medial or lateral, along the tibial crest. A corrective "Y" strip is used to surround these areas.
Addition of shock absorption material to the shoes is also helpful.

A 2 inch "I" tape, and several 1.5 to 2 inch "Y" tapes

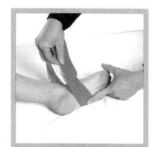

- Measure the tape length from the medial forefoot to the proximal third of the lower leg
- Anchor the "I" tape at medial aspect of arch of foot

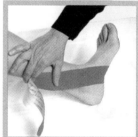

- Evert and dorsiflex the ankle as the tape is applied along the tibialis posterior muscle, with paper-off tension
- Extend the tape up the medial lower leg, along the tibialis posterior
- No tension is applied at the end of the tape

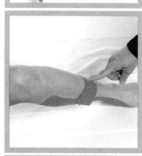

- Locate the area or areas of localized pain
- For posterior shin splints, the pain is usually along the medial tibial crest
- Anchor the "Y" tape anteriorly, just lateral to tibial crest.
- Gather fascia medial to the crest, along the painful area and support
- Lay down superior and inferior tails, surrounding pain, with moderate tension
- No tension is applied at the ends of the tails

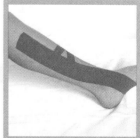

- Completed taping.
- May use several "Y" strips if pain extends up tibial crest

Ankle Dorsiflexion Assist

Tibialis Anterior
Origin: lateral surface of tibia and interosseus membrane
Insertion: plantar surface of first metatarsal and medial cuneiform
Action: dorsiflex the ankle, slight supination of the forefoot

A 2 inch "I" tape
Functional Correction

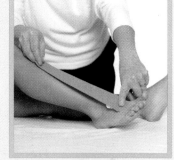

- Measure tape length from the dorsum of the foot to the proximal lower leg
- Position the leg in knee flexion and ankle dorsiflexion
- Anchor the tape on dorsum of foot
- This tape may also be anchored proximally and applied proximal to distal

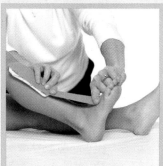

- Dorsiflex the ankle and apply second anchor to lower third of anteriolateral shin
- The amount of dorsiflexion the ankle is placed in during this application, will determine the assist the tape provides

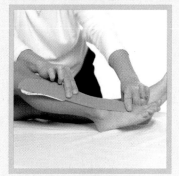

- Holding both anchors, have the child plantarflex the ankle and gently rub tape proximal to distal

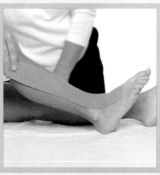

- Have the child dorsiflex ankle again, as the tape is applied up lateral shin to below knee
- This technique can be used in conjunction with the buttonhole technique, or applied with anchor at tibialis anterior, from the origin on the lateral condyle of tibia
- Completed taping for ankle dorsiflexion assist

Alternate Ankle Dorsiflexion Assist

A 2 inch "I" tape, 2 times the length of the lower leg

- Measure the tape length as twice the length of the lower leg
- Split the tape backing in the center and place the tape on plantar surface of midfoot with no tension
- Tape should be between calcaneus and metatarsal heads

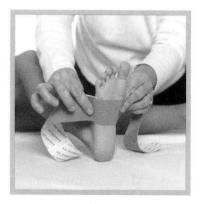

- Position the ankle in neutral alignment and dorsiflexion, with the knee flexed

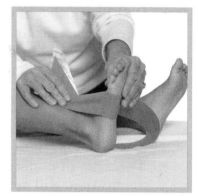

- Apply tape with paper-off tension diagonally over the anterior ankle
- Tape may be applied with increased tension on the medial section (if pronating) or the lateral section (if supinating)
- Ankle is held in neutral dorsiflexion, with knee flexed
- Tape continues up anterior lower leg with paper-off tension
- No tension is applied at the end of the tape

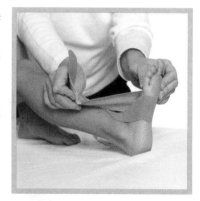

- Completed taping for ankle dorsiflexion
- This technique can be combined with other dorsiflexion assist taping techniques

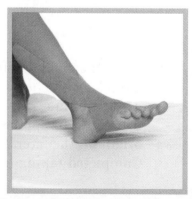

Ankle Plantarflexion Assist

This technique is a biomechanical assist, used to limit the available dorsiflexion of the ankle, as well as to support the plantarflexors. Tape may be applied origin to insertion, or insertion to origin, as the primary purpose is a mechanical assist. This technique may be used inside orthotics or splints, to assist with plantarflexion control.

Soleus
Origin: Posterior surface of head of fibula. Proximal third of posterior surface of fibula
             Soleal line and middle third of medial border of fibula
Insertion: Posterior surface of calcaneus (Achilles tendon)
Action: plantarflexes the ankle, eccentric control in stance phase of gait

Gastrocnemius
Origin: Lateral Head-Lateral condyle and posterior part of medial condyle.
             Medial Head- Proximal and posterior part of medial condyle
Insertion: near the Achilles tendon, into the middle part of the posterior surface of calcaneus.
Action: plantarflexes the ankle, flexes the knee

Two 2 inch "I" tapes

- Measure tape length from base of heel to distal knee
- Knee may be flexed or extended, as the ankle is plantarflexed
- Determine the amount of ankle plantarflexion based on the degree of plantarflexion assist required (affected also by patients height, weight, and strength, and stiffness)
- Anchor the "I" tape distal to the medial knee

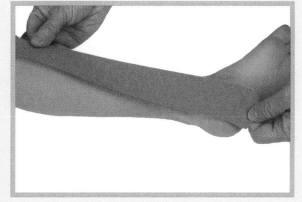

- Apply the tape with paper-off tension, along the medial gastrocnemius, and ending on the base of the calcaneus
- No tension at the end of the tape

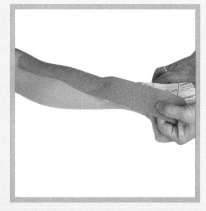

- Apply the tape with paper-off tension, along the lateral gastrocnemius and ending on the base of the calcaneus
- No tension at the end of the tape

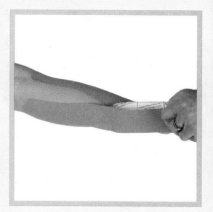

- Completed taping to assist ankle plantarflexion
- A horizontal piece of tape may be applied with no tension, along the posterior ankle horizontally, if tape pulls off

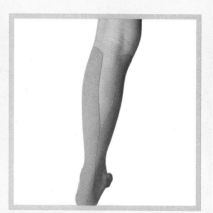

Achilles Strain

Gastrocnemius
Origin: Lateral Head-Lateral condyle and posterior part of medial condyle
                Medial Head- Proximal and posterior part of medial condyle
Insertion: near the Achilles tendon into the middle part of the posterior surface of calcaneus
Action: plantarflexion of the ankle

Soleus
Origin: Posterior surface of head of fibula. Proximal third of posterior surface of fibula
                Soleal line and middle third of medial border of fibula.
Insertion: Posterior surface of calcaneus (Achilles tendon)
Action: plantarflexion of the ankle

A 2 inch "Y" tape, a 2 inch "I" tape

- Measure the tape length from the base of the heel to just distal to the popliteal crease
- Place the child prone, with the knee extended and the ankle dorsiflexed
- Anchor the base of the "Y" under the heel

> **i** A 3 inch wide piece of tape may be used with a larger adult, or if more support is required

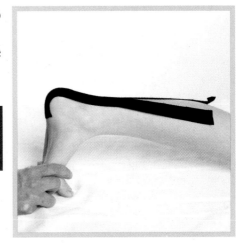

- Apply the lateral tail, with paper-off tension, along the lateral border of the gastrocnemius with the ankle in dorsiflexion
- End the tail just distal to knee, with no tension applied to the end of the tape
- Apply the medial tail, with paper-off tension, along the medial border of the gastrocnemius
- End the tail just distal to the knee with no tension applied to the end of the tape

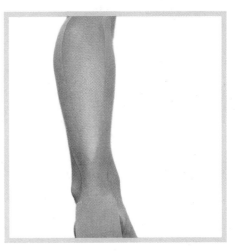

LOWER EXTREMITY

- An "I" strip may be added distal to proximal, with the ankle in dorsiflexion, to facilitate a fascial release
- A corrective strip, with full tension on the center of the tape, may be applied horizontally over the painful area of soleus or gastrocnemius

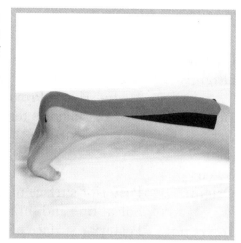

- If the child has Sever's calcaneal apophysitis or localized pain at the calcaneus; a horizontal correction strip, with full tension from the center of the tape, may be added above the calcaneus

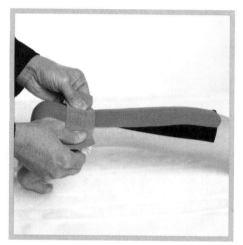

- Completed taping for Achilles tendonitis

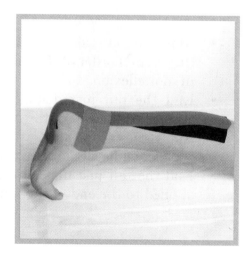

Lateral Ankle Sprain

A 2 inch "I" tape, a 2 inch "Y" tape

- Measure tape length of first piece of tape from medial hindfoot to proximal lower leg
- Measure tape length of second piece of tape from medial hindfoot to posterior heel
- Position ankle in neutral dorsiflexion and slight eversion, to protect lateral ligaments

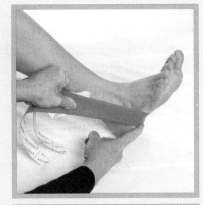

- The first piece of tape is anchored under the medial hindfoot, anterior to the calcaneus
- Tape is applied with paper-off tension under the heel
- Moderate to maximal tension is applied to the tape as it crosses the lateral ankle
- Tape tails are applied up lateral lower leg with paper-off tension
- No tension is applied at the end of the tape

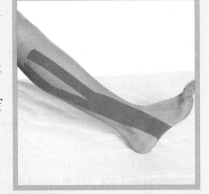

- The second piece of tape is anchored under the medial hindfoot, anterior to the calcaneus
- Tape is applied with paper-off tension under the heel
- Moderate to maximal tension is applied to the tape as it crosses the lateral heel on a diagonal
- No tension is applied at the end of the tape, as it wraps around the posterior heel

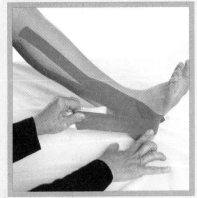

- Completed taping for a lateral ankle sprain
- This technique may be combined with taping for swelling and edema
- More support is added by overlapping tape over the tape
- A third piece of tape may also be added, extending over the anterio-lateral ankle
- This tape may be worn under rigid tape with underwrap, which may be added for additional support during increased activity

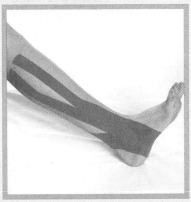

Foot Pronation

A thorough evaluation of lower extremity biomechanical alignment need to be completed in order to properly asses the causative factors in foot pronation. (Cusick)

- Often proximal malalignment issues (i.e. increased medial femoral torsion, genu varum) contribute to ankle and foot position.
- Know bony alignment and developmental norms.
- Know how to assess ankle and foot mobility, range of motion, alignment and subtalar neutral position.
- Taping is often combined with orthotics for optimal alignment.
- Can be done in prone (preferred) or sitting

Technique 1: Prone
3 or 4 "I" tapes, 2 inches wide

Foot Alignment/Stabilization
Evaluate:
- Ankle range of motion
- Subtalar neutral
- Calcaneal inversion/eversion
- Leg varum and relaxed calcaneal stance for relaxed eversion angle
- Forefoot alignment (varus/valgus)
- First ray position and mobility

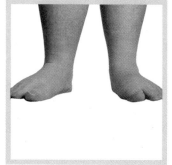 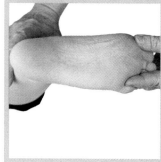

- For a pronated foot: place foot in subtalar neutral position, or minimal inversion and neutral dorsiflexion
- Anchor the first piece of tape on the lateral midfoot and bring the tape diagonally under calcaneus and medially around posterior ankle
- The tape is applied with paper-off tension, unless additional support is required. If this is the case, increased tension may be applied to the center of the tape

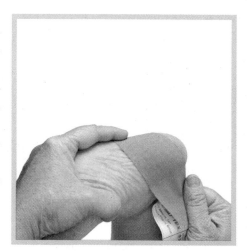

- This piece of tape will help maintain calcaneus in a more neutral position and limit calcaneal eversion

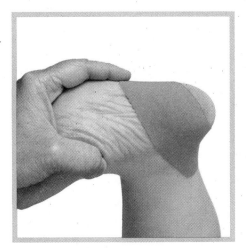

- Anchor the second piece of tape on medial midfoot and bring diagonally under calcaneus and laterally around posterior ankle
- Be sure to maintain neutral or slightly inverted position of calcaneus
- Tape functions to assist to "lock" calcaneus in position or "close the loop" for sensory input

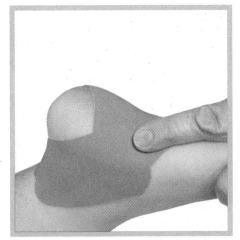

- The third piece of tape extends from the lateral midfoot, over navicular and up the medial distal third of the lower leg, just above the malleolus
- The tape is applied with paper-off tension and the ankle is positioned in subtalar neutral position
- This tape supports the midfoot

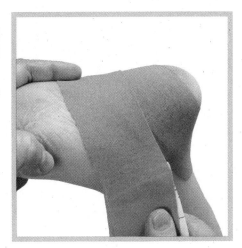

- A second piece of tape can be applied over or overlapping the first for more support
- Additional tension can also be applied along medial deltoid ligament for more support

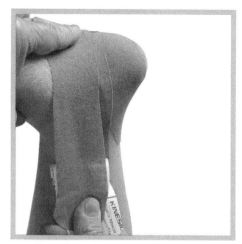

- A fourth piece of tape may be added to "create" a peroneus longus and assist to bring the first ray down
- Anchor the tape on dorsum of first metatarsal head and plantarflex first ray as you bring tape diagonally under foot and up over lateral malleolus with paper-off tension. This functions as a mechanical hold
- No tension is applied at the end of the tape

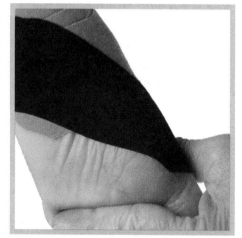

- Tape can also be applied from origin to insertion to facilitate peroneus longus. Remember to plantarflex the first ray for application
- Completed taping for foot pronation

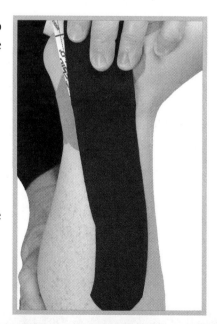

- This piece of tape will help maintain calcaneus in a more neutral position and limit calcaneal eversion

- For a pronated foot: place in subtalar neutral position, or minimal inversion and neutral dorsiflexion
- Anchor the first piece of tape on the lateral midfoot and bring the tape diagonally under calcaneus and medially around posterior ankle
- The tape is applied with paper-off tension, unless additional support is required. If this is the case, increased tension may be applied to the center of the tape
- This piece of tape will help maintain calcaneus in a more neutral position and limit calcaneal eversion

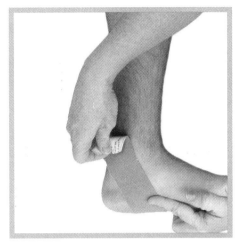

- Anchor the second piece of tape on medial midfoot and bring diagonally under calcaneus and laterally around posterior ankle
- Be sure to maintain neutral or slightly inverted position of calcaneus
- Tape functions to assist to "lock" calcaneus in position or "close the loop" for sensory input

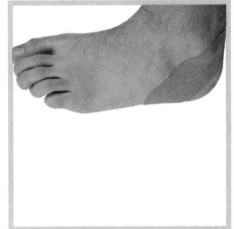

- The third piece of tape extends from the lateral midfoot, over navicular and up the medial distal third of lower leg, just above the malleolus
- The tape is applied with paper-off tension and the ankle is positioned in subtalar neutral position
- This tape supports the midfoot

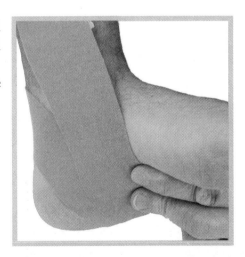

LOWER EXTREMITY

- A second piece of tape can be applied over or overlapping the first for more support
- Additional tension can also be applied along medial deltoid ligament for more support

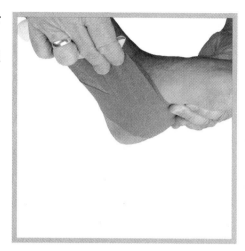

- A fourth piece of tape may be added to "create" a peroneus longus and assist to bring the first ray down
- Anchor the tape on dorsum of first metatarsal head and plantarflex first ray as you bring tape diagonally under foot and up over lateral malleolus with paper-off tension. This functions as a mechanical hold
- No tension is applied at the end of the tape
- Tape can also be applied from origin to insertion to facilitate peroneus longus. Remember to plantarflex the first ray for application

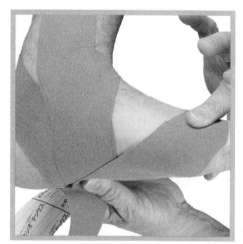

- Completed taping for foot pronation

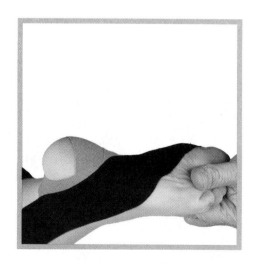

Foot Supination

A thorough evaluation of lower extremity biomechanical alignment need to be completed in order to properly assess the causative factors in foot supination. (Cusick)
- Often proximal malalignment issues (i.e. increased medial femoral torsion, genu varum) contribute to ankle and foot position.
- Know bony alignment and developmental norms.
- Know how to assess ankle and foot mobility, range of motion, alignment and subtalar neutral position.
- Taping is often combined with orthotics for optimal alignment.

3 or 4 "I" tapes, 2 inches wide

Foot Alignment/Stabilization
Evaluate:
- Ankle range of motion
- Subtalar neutral
- Calcaneal inversion/eversion
- Leg varum and relaxed calcaneal stance for relaxed eversion angle
- Forefoot alignment (varus/valgus)
- First ray position and mobility

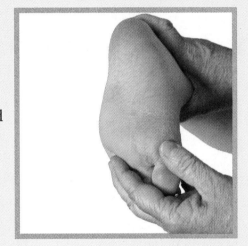

- For a supinated foot: place foot in subtalar neutral position, or minimal eversion and neutral dorsiflexion
- Anchor the first piece of tape on the medial midfoot and bring the tape diagonally under calcaneus and laterally around posterior ankle

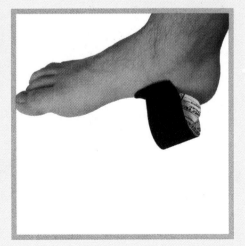

- The tape is applied with paper-off tension, unless additional support is required. If this is the case, increased tension may be applied to the center of the tape
- This piece of tape will help maintain calcaneus in a more neutral position and limit calcaneal inversion

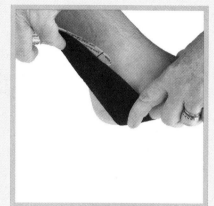

Optional:
- Anchor the second piece of tape on lateral midfoot and bring diagonally under calcaneus and medially around posterior ankle
- Be sure to maintain neutral or slightly everted position of calcaneus
- Tape functions to assist to "lock" calcaneus in position and provide sensory input

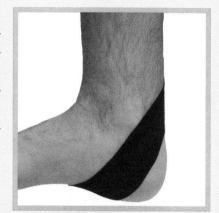

- The third piece of tape extends from the medial midfoot to the plantar surface and over the styloid to the distal third of lower leg
- The tape is applied with paper-off tension and the ankle is positioned in subtalar neutral position or slight eversion
- This tape supports the midfoot

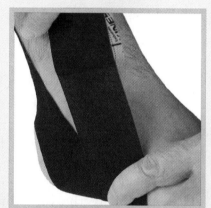

- Completed foot pronation taping
- Observe position at rest and in weight bearing, as indicated

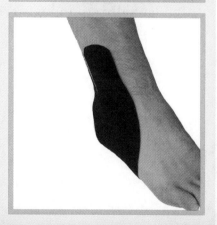

Metatarsus Adductus

Three 1.5 or 2 inch "I" tapes

- Assess and measure forefoot adduction
- Bisect the heel and bisect the forefoot
- Measure the position at rest, as well as the amount of forefoot abduction available
- Measure tape length from base of 5th metatarsal to the medial midfoot

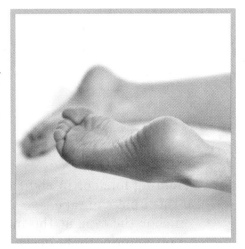

- Anchor tape at the 5th metatarsal head
- Hold the forefoot in as much abduction as available, using moderate force, depending on child's age
- Pull full tension out of the tape, as it is applied to the lateral border of the foot

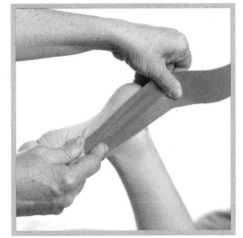

- Apply the tape with paper-off tension coming around heel to the medial foot
- Reassess foot alignment and position after taping
- May add a second piece of tape, using same technique, overlapping the first piece to provide a stronger pull

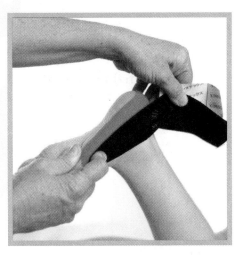

- Reassess the foot alignment and position again, to determine if it has improved

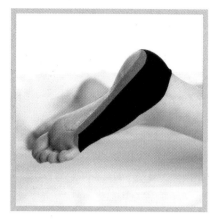

- Holding forefoot in abduction and slight eversion, apply a third piece of tape
- Anchor the tape at the medial midfoot and continue to apply anterior to the heel and to lateral leg, over malleolus, with paper-off tension
- No tension is applied at the end of the tape

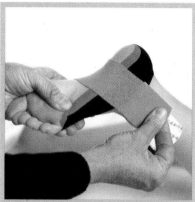

- Completed taping: lateral view

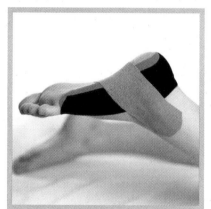

- Completed taping: medial view

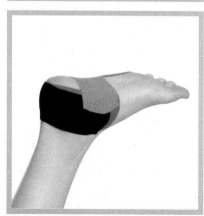

Kinesio Taping® in Pediatrics

Plantar Fascitis

Plantar Fascitis is an inflammation of the plantar aponeurosis. Pain and inflammation are generally felt at the origin on the anterior aspect of the calcaneus. Range of motion in the plantar fascia and gastrocnemius and soleus need to be assessed. Decreased range of motion into ankle dorsiflexion may contribute to plantar fascitis.

A 2 or 3 inch fan tape, a 2 inch "I" tape

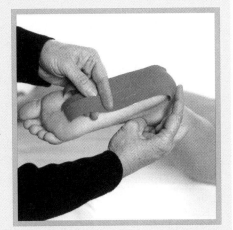

- Measure the entire length of from the metatarsal heads to approximately 2 inches above the musculotendinous junction of the gastrocnemius and Achilles
- On one end, cut a 4 or 5 strip-fan tape, extending from the metatarsal heads to the calcaneal tubercle
- Anchor the tape on the posterior heel and apply with paper-off tension to the base of the calcaneus

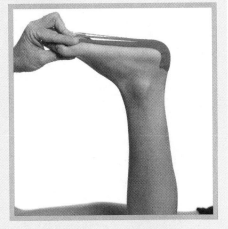

- Keeping the foot in dorsiflexion, apply full tension on one of the 5 tails which have been cut
- Place this strip from the calcaneus to the space between the first and second ray (toe) on the metatarsal head.
- Continue the same process by placing a strip of Kinesio® Tex tape between the second and third, third and fourth, and fourth and fifth toes
- A space between the plantar surface of the foot and the tape should be present

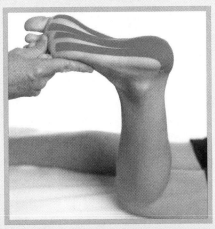

- Provide pressure through the plantar surface of the foot as you rub the tape to distribute the support of the Kinesio® Tape
- Trim edges of tape at metatarsal heads, to end at metatarsal heads

- Optional: A horizontal piece of tape may be applied, with no tension, to hold ends of tape if tape begins to peel off

- The second piece of tape supports the metatarsal arch
- Place the foot in neutral
- Anchor the "I" strip, with no tension, near the base of the 5th metatarsal on the lateral aspect of the foot

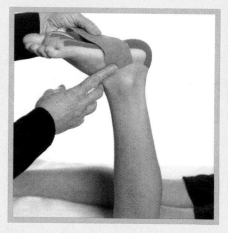

- The tape is angled to support the midtarsal arch and the application continues over the medial aspect of the foot and lower leg with paper-off tension on the plantar surface and extend up medial arch with moderate tension

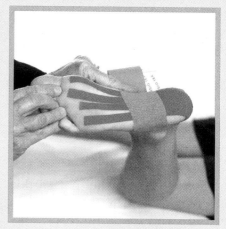

- Completed taping for plantar fascitis

i This technique may be combined with the technique for an Achilles strain, during acute inflammation

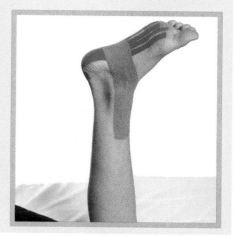

Hallux Valgus

Technique 1:
 A 2 inch fan cut, with hole cut into proximal third, near anchor

- Anchor tape on dorsum of first metatarsal head
- The base of the donut hole strip is placed superior to the first MCP joint
- The hole is placed over the first MCP joint, with moderate tension
- The first ray may be rotated laterally and abducted slightly as the tape is applied

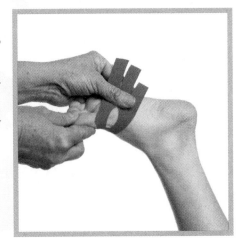

- The three tails are applied on plantar surface of foot, with no tension on the plantar surface of the foot

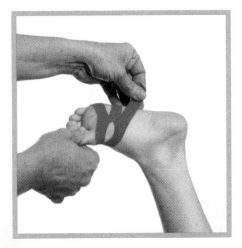

- Completed taping for hallux valgus

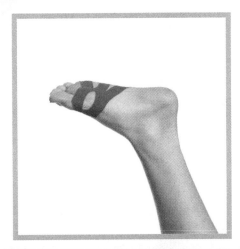

Technique 2: A 2 inch "Y" strip

- Measure tape length from nail bed of the first toe to the hindfoot, medially
- Place the base of a "Y" strip on the DIP of the great toe, with the split in the "Y" cut just distal to the first metatarsophalangeal joint

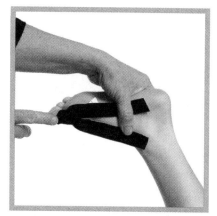

- The superior tail is applied slightly above the first ray, with moderate tension
- No tension is applied at the end of the tape

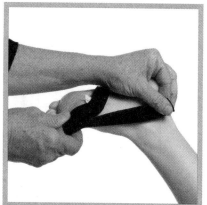

- Apply moderate tension to the inferior strip, with the tail running slightly below the first ray
- The first toe may be abducted slightly as tape is applied.
- No tension is applied to either the beginning or end of the "Y" strip
- This may be modified by using two 1 inch Kinesio® Tex "I" pieces of tape

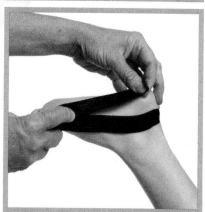

- Completed taping for hallux valgus
- Both techniques may be combined

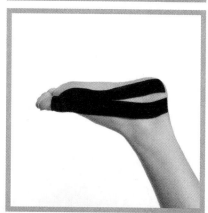

Toe Clawing

Toe clawing is a normal developmental phase infants go through, often when they first begin to stand. Toe clawing is also seen in children with sensory processing disorder and children with CNS involvement. This technique is beneficial to help to relax the toe flexors. In working with children with hypersensitivity, it is important to prepare the sensory system prior to taping. This can be accomplished with tactile input to the body, and specifically the lower extremity.

Toe Extensors:
Origin: fibula and interosseus membrane
Insertion: first to fifth toes
Action: extends the toes

Tibialis Anterior
Origin: lateral surface of tibia & interosseus membrane
Insert: plantar surface of 1st metatarsal & medial cuneiform
Action: dorsiflex ankle, slight supination of foot

A 2 or 3 inch "I" tape with diamond-shaped cutouts for toes

- Measure the tape length to cover the bottom of the foot and the dorsum of the foot, extending up lower leg
- Fold tape over and cut 3-4 triangle shapes (to be diamond shapes) for the toes
- Tear the backing from the center of the diamonds and gently peel and fold back the edges

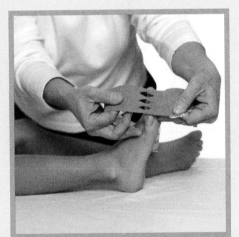

- Gently place each diamond cut between the toes, and anchor with no tension on dorsum and plantar surface of the foot

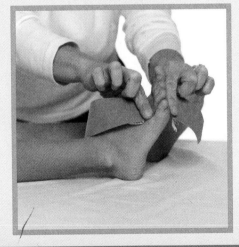

- Place the ankle in dorsiflexion and anchor the tape on the lower leg
- Plantarflex the ankle and adhere tape
- Apply the tape to the leg with paper-off tension
- No tension is applied at either end of the tape

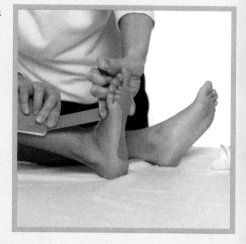

- Completed taping for toe clawing
- This technique may be done with ankle in neutral position for proprioceptive input

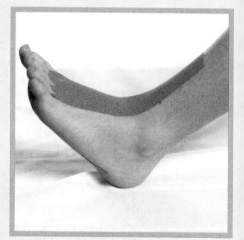

- This technique may be combined with a dorsiflexion assist taping, as one piece of tape, or as a separate

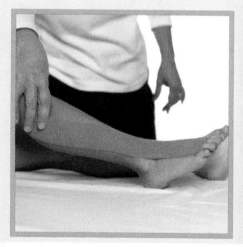

DIAGNOSIS SPECIFIC TAPING

Low Tone

Jamie is a young boy with a diagnosis of Down Syndrome. He exhibits overall decreased postural control against gravity. Jamie is hypotonic and displays hypermobility at the wrists, fingers and thumb metacarpal phalangeal joints, as well as in his hips, knees and ankles. He demonstrates difficulty with grading his movement for speed and control. His equilibrium reactions are delayed in standing and he uses a wide base of support in stance. Jamie is able to run and ascend and descend stairs independently.

This is Jamie's typical standing posture. He tends to stand and walk with a wide base of support. His lower extremities are positioned in lateral rotation and his upper extremities are positioned in shoulder internal rotation.

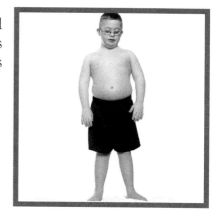

Jamie exhibits decreased postural stability, with an increase in his sacral angle secondary to poor active control of his abdominals.

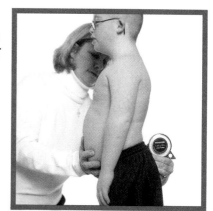

This is Jamie's posture prior to abdominal taping.

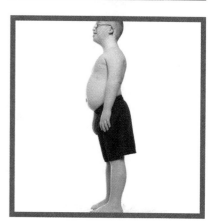

Kinesio® Tape was applied to the internal and external abdominal obliques and transversus abdominis.

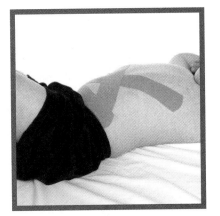

After taping the abdominals there was a decrease in his sacral angle.

Jamie's center of gravity also moved posteriorly, as he used his abdominals and gluteals to shift his weight. His knees are slightly flexed, and his ankles in more dorsiflexion.

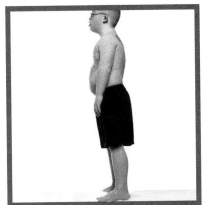

Poor proximal stabilization of the shoulder girdle may interfere with graded reaching.

Jamie's scapula was positioned "down and in" into more optimal alignment. He was cued to maintain a more upright posture.

Kinesio® Tape was applied, taping the lower trapezius by anchoring the "I" tape at T12 and laying down the tape with paper off tension.

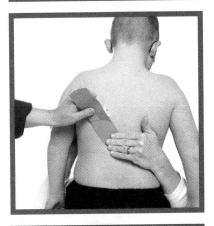

The tape was applied toward the acromion with paper off tension while Jamie maintained scapular alignment.

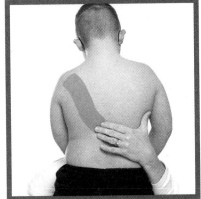

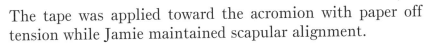

The middle trapezius was taped by anchoring tape at the spinous processes of T2-T3 and laying down tape with paper off tension in a horizontal direction, along the spine of the scapula.

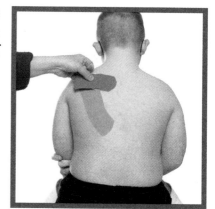

Stabilizing the scapula in combination with the abdominals, will assist with the development of proximal stability of the trunk.

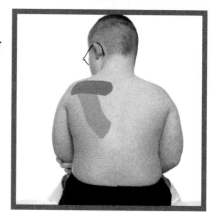

This taping technique was applied bilaterally to improve Jamie's shoulder girdle stability.

The incorporation of exercises to strengthen the abdominals and scapular musculature is important in the therapy program.

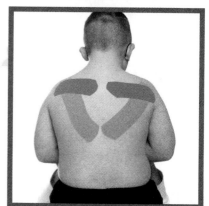

Kinesio® Tape was then applied to decrease pronation.

As proximal control improves and base of support decreases, weight will be shifted more laterally on Jamie's feet.

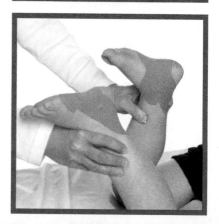

Completed taping.

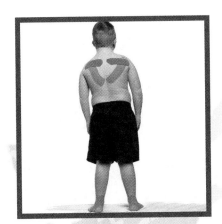

Position before taping

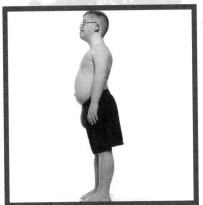

Position after taping

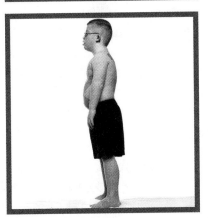

Stability through taping may assist with execution of graded and efficient movement.

Graded muscle control may be developed through the facilitation of weightshifting through the trunk and pelvis. Controlled movement requires postural stability and a strong core as an anchor for dynamic movement.

Balance may be further developed through closed chain weightbearing activities involving lower extremities.

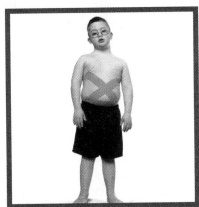

Hemiplegia

Prior assessment of a child with CNS dysfunction is essential to prioritize effective taping and treatment planning. The achievement of optimal musculoskeletal alignment is important for functional performance. It is essential to identify the area to be taped and the therapeutic intervention that can best be used to achieve optimal motor control.

Bonnie is a nine year old girl with a diagnosis of right hemiplegia. Bonnie has not had any orthopedic surgeries and is involved in occupational and physical therapy with a strong home program of stretching, strengthening, electrical stimulation and taping. The following is a brief synopsis of her posture.

In standing, Bonnie tends to keep her weight shifted toward her uninvolved side with an anteriorly tilted pelvis. She has a slight leg length discrepancy, right lower extremity 1.5 cm shorter than the left and right hip retraction. She also has bilateral genu recurvatum with the left greater than the right and bilateral ankle pronation. She ambulates independently and is able to use a heel-toe gait pattern on the right. Her step length on the right is only slightly shorter than the left. Bonnie has been taped for facilitation of hip lateral rotation, abdominal obliques and gluteus maximus. She has also been taped to decrease knee hyperextension and ankle pronation.

She has slight shortening of the right trunk. Her right scapula is in downward rotation with the inferior border tipped out and the right shoulder rotated medially. Movement of the right upper extremity is initiated with shoulder elevation, humeral abduction, and left lateral tilting of the trunk. Bonnie demonstrates difficultly with end range shoulder flexion and abduction overhead. To initiate this movement, she positions the humerus into internal rotation with shortening of the pectoralis major and minor. When reaching, she tends to position her forearm in pronation, which biomechanically places her distal arm in wrist flexion, ulnar deviation and thumb flexion.

Bonnie is independent with basic self care, requiring extra time for tasks involving bilateral hand manipulation. She uses an immature mass grasp and release pattern with difficulty incorporating her thumb for prehension. Bonnie typically uses a gross lateral pinch for grasp. She demonstrates active finger flexion and extension with her wrist positioned into flexion. The wrist extensors are weak and she is unable to extend her wrist and fingers simultaneously. Bonnie is able to reach for items overhead or in front of her body with the right hand along with compensatory trunk movements. She has undergone serial casting to her right upper extremity and taping for scapular stabilization, and facilitation of forearm supination, wrist extension, and radial deviation.

Therapy goals include the achievement of optimal musculoskeletal alignment prior to facilitating movement in the treatment session. Kinesio® Taping techniques are utilized to achieve this goal. Once new muscle length and alignment have been achieved, Bonnie is challenged to use this alignment actively during functional daily tasks.

Observe Bonnie's resting posture and the position of her shoulder girdle and trunk.
Note her forward right shoulder, downwardly rotated scapula with the inferior border tipped, and slight shortening of her right trunk.

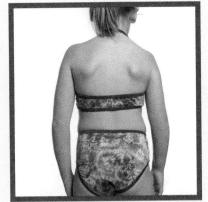

Kinesio® Tex tape was applied to stabilize the right scapula onto the thoracic wall and facilitate muscle action by taping the lower and middle trapezius. Taping for the forward posture to bring the shoulder "back and down" into alignment was also utilized.

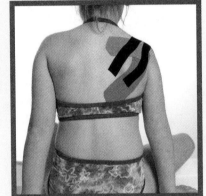

At rest, her forearm is in pronation, with the wrist flexed and thumb adducted. The pronated forearm biomechanically influences the position of her hand for prehension. It will be difficult for her to grasp items without forearm supination and wrist extension.

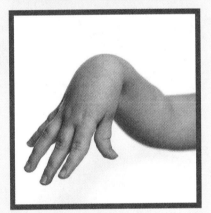

Bonnie was taped for supination to align the forearm position and wrist extension to support the weak wrist. Thumb extension taping was applied to position the thumb and wrist in a more neutral alignment.
With continued therapy a palmar stability taping technique can be applied to facilitate thumb finger prehension.

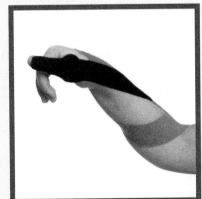

In standing, her scapula and humerus are in a more optimal alignment and her palm is facing her thigh.

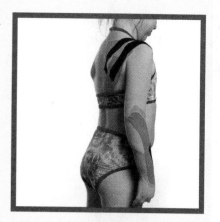

Bonnie's base of support will influence the alignment of her upper extremity.

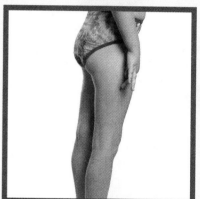

Her right leg is slightly shorter than left. The left knee is in recurvatum and both ankles are in pronation.

Abdominal taping and/or taping to decrease recurvatum could be utilized as well.

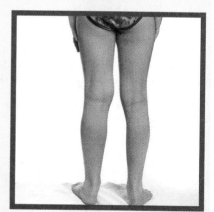

Kinesio® Tape is applied to bring the calcaneus into a more neutral position and to support the midtarsal joint. Tape is also used to facilitate the peroneus longus and bringing the first ray down.

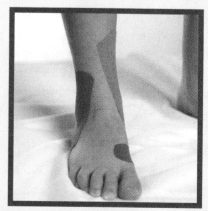

The calcaneus is positioned in more neutral alignment with decreased eversion. The calcaneus is supported medially and laterally for stability.

A thorough lower extremity biomechanical assessment is key to determine appropriate taping intervention.

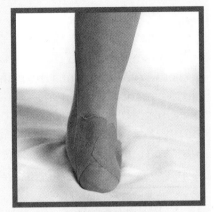

Position before taping

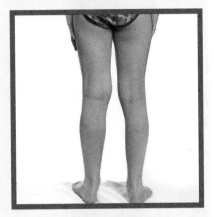

Position after taping

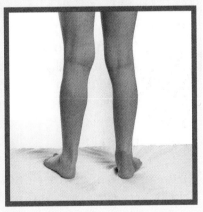

Bobby is a 6 week old baby boy with right obstetric brachial plexus injury. As a result, Bobby presents with partial paralysis of his right arm and shoulder girdle. The poor alignment and posturing of the right arm reflect the muscle imbalance occurring as a result of the nerve injury. It is important to evaluate Bobby in sitting, supine, and prone and to observe resting position and spontaneous movements in both arms. This observation of Bobby's movements will provide information of the muscle activity as an indication of innervation. Lack of movement may indicate decreased or absent innervation or disuse atrophy in muscles that are now innervated.

To identify areas to be taped, it is important to understand the sequence of the developmental motor milestones. There are numerous courses and references on the subject of normal development. To identify areas of motor weakness or abnormal sensorimotor development, it is necessary to clinically observe the motor patterns, muscle contraction and movement components which make each developmental milestone possible. At this age, knowledge and observation of age appropriate reflexes is essential, as well as assessment of asymmetries.

Bobby exhibits the classic posturing seen in infants with an upper brachial plexus palsy (waiter's tip). This presents as an adducted, medially rotated shoulder, extended elbow, pronated forearm, flexed and ulnarly deviated wrist with fingers and thumb in flexion. Bobby tends to use stronger muscles for reach and these compensatory movements may become a learned pattern for function. As the nerves regenerate, atrophy in muscles and inability to coordinate movement need to be assessed. Taping techniques should target specific muscles with results carefully monitored to ensure optimal alignment in movement. For example, in selecting the muscles for function, taping the wrist in neutral deviation and extension, forearm supination, elbow flexion and external rotation of the humerus may assist with bringing the hand to mouth. Kinesio® Tape can be applied to provide optimal alignment, assist the desired muscle activity and to decrease compensatory movement. An example of a compensatory movement is the use of the middle deltoid with the shoulder internally rotated and elevated for Bobby to bring his hand to his mouth.

To ensure optimal function, the prevention of soft tissue contractures and sensory neglect of the arm is key. Kinesio® Taping may provide proprioceptive input to assist with the development of the child's awareness of the arm and hand. In addition, the colored Kinesio® Tape will provide increased visual awareness. The neglect of the arm may be a factor secondary to decreased sensory awareness and poor motor control. After application of Kinesio® Tape, careful evaluation and training of Bobby's functional movement patterns needs to be assessed and monitored. Potential improvement may be facilitated by encouraging Bobby to practice movement in more optimal alignment, with Kinesio® Tape assisting.

At six weeks, when placed in sitting, Bobby begins to gain extension control over physiological flexion.

The asymmetrical tonic neck reflex (ATNR) has strong influence on posturing of the extremities.

If his trunk is supported, Bobby may extend his head and thoracic spine, but will not be able to grade this movement. This is developmentally appropriate.

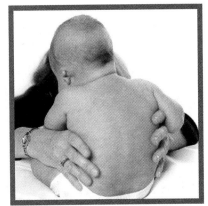

In prone Bobby is able to clear his head and shows active neck rotation with extension. As he lifts and turns his head, his weight is transferred to his arms and shoulders. The majority of body weight in prone is on the upper extremities and head, secondary to the elevated position of the pelvis and the hip flexion contractures normally present at this age.

Bobby has minimal shoulder girdle stability, with his left wrist in neutral and hand fisted. Bobby's right wrist is in flexion with wrist in ulnar deviation and fingers flexed.

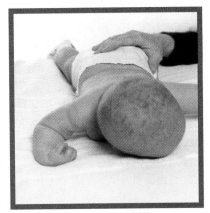

In prone, Bobby exhibits shoulder elevation bilaterally. The rotator cuff muscles are active and support the shoulders. His upper extremity weightbearing occurs primarily at the shoulder, forearm and base of the hand. His elbow is positioned behind his shoulder on the left.

Following myofascial release to the right arm, the Kinesio® Tape is applied with the buttonhole technique. The tape is placed between his fingers to provide palmar input and stability, as well as to improve wrist extension and forearm supination. This position allows input to the ulnar side of the hand and enables Bobby to use the surface of the floor to stabilize his arm.

Taping is followed by a functional activity in this alignment.

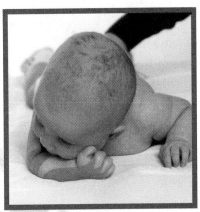

In supine, Bobby can randomly move his uninvolved left arm into shoulder abduction, adduction, and flexion. The left arm is abducted and externally rotated, with gravity and movement assisting to lengthen the pectoralis major and minor muscles. Bobby is able to flex and extend at his left elbow.

Weakness in his right involved arm makes it difficult for Bobby to bring his hand to mouth. His arm is held at his side, with elbow extended and he has difficulty moving his right arm against gravity.

By placing rolled towels under his shoulder girdle, the right

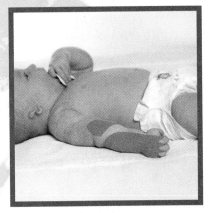

shoulder can be supported forward to facilitate elbow flexion in Bobby's visual field. Bobby is able to gaze at his hand during movement. It is important to encourage hand to mouth, hand to hand, and to develop midline control at an age appropriate time.

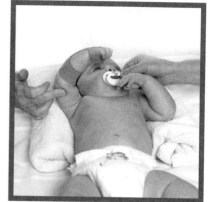

In prone, Bobby uses asymmetrical neck and trunk extension to lift his head. As his head is lifted, Bobby pushes into the surface with his left arm abducted. Scapular abduction and adduction are beginning to develop as scapular stability increases.

In prone, the tape assists to position right arm, facilitating input into the right involved arm. Elongation of the ulnar side of the wrist occurs as Bobby brings his hand to his mouth.

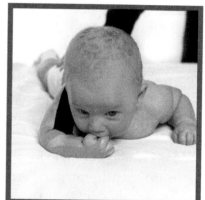

In side lying, movements in a small controlled range are available, especially hand to hand, hand to mouth and midline activities.

This position can be used to assist Bobby in use of his right arm more effectively, as gravity is eliminated.

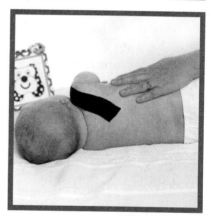

In sitting, Bobby has increased shoulder elevation of his involved arm. Bobby has decreased scapular stability on the right, and uses his upper trapezius to try to stabilize against gravity. Kinesio® Tape could also be applied to lower and middle trapezius to facilitate shoulder depression. Prioritize taping applications, to limit input and allow Bobby to integrate new alignment and control gradually.

Completed taping for this infant's brachial plexus injury

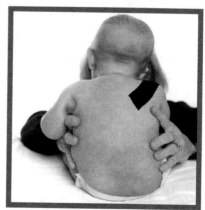

The Use of Kinesio® Tape in the Treatment of Torticollis

The term torticollis is derived from the Latin words "torti" meaning twisted, and "collum" for neck. Congenital muscular torticollis refers to a condition caused by idiopathic fibrosis of the sternocleidomastoid muscle that restricts movement and pulls the head toward the involved side and rotates toward the opposite side. (Yu et al, 2004)

Positional torticollis is a term used to define asymmetric head position, often accompanied by plagiocephaly. These two types of torticollis, as well as associated concerns, are reviewed with accompanying suggestions for the use of Kinesio® Tex tape applications as an adjunct to treatment.

The asymmetric tonic neck reflex is dominant in infants and often not fully integrated until the child is six months old. Midline control does not typically develop until nearly three months of age.

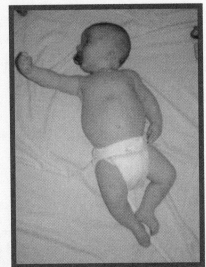

When infants spend a great deal of time in supine, they are unable to maintain midline position, and tend to turn their heads in one direction. This is exacerbated by the influence of the ATNR reflex.

Congenital muscular torticollis (CMT) is most commonly seen in infants under one year of age, though has been documented in older children. CMT responds well to therapy in over ninety percent of the cases. The incidence is about 0.4-1.9% and is greater in males and on the right, as opposed to the left sternocleidomastoid. It is also more commonly seen in breech deliveries. The etiology of CMT is questionable with possible causes including compartment syndrome from in-utero positioning, muscle kinking during delivery, ischemic injury to muscle, nerve and muscle injury, swelling, and fibrous tissue replacement (Davides et al 1993).

Differential diagnosis includes consideration of several issues: (Semen, Conway 2000)
Vertebral anomaly (30%)
Ocular involvement (23%)
Brachial plexus injury (17%)
Neurologic involvement (11%)
Gastroesophageal reflux, pharyngitis, Sandifer syndrome, and benign paroxysmal torticollis also need to be considered.
Torticollis can be an isolated deformity or a sign of other neuromuscular disease.
(Wolfert et al 1989)

Secondary complications occur with both congenital muscular torticollis and positional torticollis. Postural asymmetries with compensatory movement patterns will affect development and alignment and cause further mobility issues. Diminished strength in the over lengthened muscles will affect grading of movement in all planes. Asymmetrical weight shifts will impact the entire body as the infant and child learn to move.

In the assessment of torticollis, many factors need to be considered. A complete pregnancy and birth history is essential. Assessment of range of motion, eye movements, skeletal asymmetries and neurologic status needs to be included. The infant or child needs to be undressed, to look at joint position and range of motion in the whole body. The presence of an SCM fibrotic nodule may be found in congenital muscular torticollis. This nodule develops in approximately one-half to two-thirds of children diagnosed with CMT. It may appear between two to four weeks of age and grow larger for a few months, until it gradually resolves. Fibrotic tissue does not grow proportionately and may cause further shortening of the SCM.

Cranial molding also occurs, as a result of the pressure of the floor or surface on the cranial bones and flattening of one side is often observed. This is accompanied by a rounding at the occiput, making it even more difficult for the infant to turn his or her head or maintain midline. The initiation of the "Back to Sleep" campaign launched in 1994 to decrease the incidence of Sudden Infant Death Syndrome in infants may be correlated with an increase in plagiocephaly. Use of infant seats and car seats has increased as parents are "on the go" and gravity works to hold infants head to one side or the other. When infants sleep in one position, there is consistent pressure on their soft and forming skull, which can result in deformation of the head. (Graham, 1999) It is important for pediatricians and parents to recognize the importance of midline positioning and "tummy time" in prone.

Plagiocephaly is often observed in infants with torticollis and must be evaluated. Congenital muscular torticollis or positional torticollis causing an SCM imbalance both indicate SCM dysfunction and may act as a precursor to positional plagiocephaly and should be treated at the earliest opportunity. (Golden et al, 1999) In torticollis, it is common to observe associated ipsilateral fronto-orbital flattening and contralateral parieto-occipital flattening.

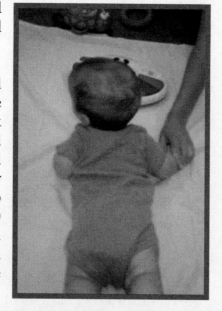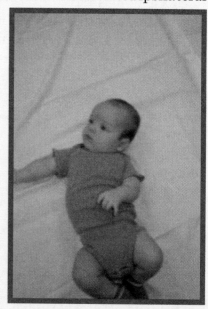

Deformation of the craniofacial skeleton will develop if the restriction of CMT is not corrected. Three dimensional computed tomography was used to evaluate craniofacial deformity in fourteen patients aged one to twenty-four. (Yu et al, 2004) Results showed that cranium and cranial base deformation took place in infancy, with the most prominent change in the posterior cranial fossa. Facial bone asymmetry appeared after five years, with mandible and occlusal abnormalities. Deformity of orbits and maxilla occurred at an older age. Craniofacial asymmetry is present in ninety percent of the children diagnosed with CMT.

The use of Kinesio® Tex tape can be beneficial to assist in facilitating overlengthened muscles and promoting optimal alignment in infants and children with torticollis. Kinesio® Tape is applied to the over lengthened SCM muscle, origin to insertion (medial clavicle to mastoid), on infants with torticollis. It has been this therapist's experience that Kinesio® Tape applied to the overlengthened SCM from mastoid to clavicle (insertion to origin) may be more effective in children over six months. The rationale for this can include the sensory input from the tape, facilitating the SCM. Input from the visual system also orients to midline and the head may be considered a functional origin in aligning posture to upright and providing midline orientation.

Range of motion in soft tissue of the tight SCM, scalenes, splenius capitus, upper trapezius, and fascial system need to be facilitated prior to taping the overlengthened muscles. Tape may be applied to the upper trapezius, from insertion to origin in the lengthened position (acromion to mastoid and horizontal to spinous process of scapula). Kinesio® Tex tape can also be applied to facilitate lower and middle trapezius. Addressing scapular position using facilitation of the middle and lower trapezius may be more beneficial, as often soft tissue massage is done in the shortened upper trapezius area and tape would limit ability to work directly on the skin.

Often in pediatrics, Kinesio® Tex tape is applied with muscles to be facilitated in a more neutral, as opposed to lengthened position, especially in children with neurological involvement and/or significant muscle imbalances. In taping the SCM, the tape is applied initially with the SCM in a lengthened position, as the input is so strong that even this may facilitate rotation to the opposite side and lateral bend toward the same side. After tape application, position should be assessed. It is important not to attempt to progress too quickly and provide too much tension on the tape as, the muscles will fatigue and tolerance will be decreased. Older children, who are up against gravity most of the day, will fatigue more quickly.

In taping for torticollis, look at SCM for tightness, look at scapulae for asymmetry, and look at upper trapezius for tightness/shoulder elevation. After assessing skin tolerance to tape with a small patch on the upper thoracic area, tape the scapula first to stabilize, after mobilizing.

Taping techniques most often used include the following:

Lower trapezius and middle trapezius facilitation (on shortened side):

Look at opposite side for guidance. Scapulae do not descend until until two months of age.

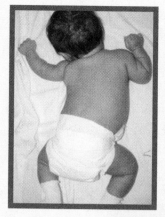
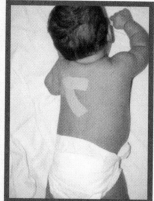

Upper trapezius relaxation: (on the shortened side, though may not be indicated as limited soft tissue massage over this area).

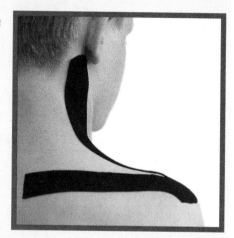

Sternocleidomastoid: (on the over lengthened side)

Tape weak SCM in a lengthened position, after assuring there is range past midline in the tight SCM, neck extensors, and scalenes. Tape the overlengthened SCM.

Anterior Scalene: (on the over lengthened side)

Kinesio® Tex tape may also be applied to the overlengthened scalene muscles if an asymmetric head tilt is evident. Tape can be applied from trunk to head. As deep neck flexors are not well-developed, taping anterior scalene alone is often indicated.

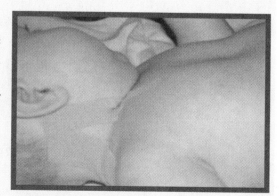

DIAGNOSIS SPECIFIC TAPING

Combination scalene and SCM taping:

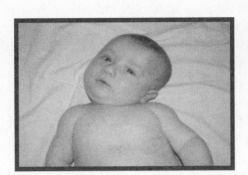 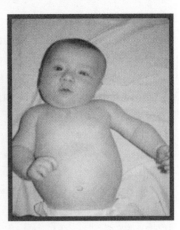

Taping Techniques:

- Initially apply a tape patch to the infant/child's upper back area to assess for skin reaction or irritability. A barrier (such as Milk of Magnesia) may need to be applied under the tape. Caregivers remove gently after 4-5 days and assess skin condition. This accompanies stretching exercises and scapular mobilization. A cervical spine x-ray may be indicated as well and should be discussed with the pediatrician.
- Taping of upper trapezius to lengthen, or middle/lower trapezius to facilitate scapular stability and shoulder depression may be indicated. Functional activities to facilitate active shoulder depression, head righting, neck rotation, and weightshift should be initiated with stretching.
- Taping of overlengthened SCM and/or scalenes is indicated once range of motion and mobility past neutral have been achieved. Use of cut-out foam wedge, soft collar, TOT collar (once upright), may also be used.
- Assessment for cranial banding or helmeting may also be indicated.
- Tape is worn for 4-6 days weekly and placement may change with each application. Constant monitoring of skin integrity is essential.
- Taping to facilitate abdominals may also be beneficial.

Early detection and intervention is key to the treatment of CMT and positional torticollis. Treatment needs to continue beyond the achievement of SCM mobility. Children need to be followed from infancy until at least one year of age. Cervical lengthening will cause head tilt to increase, often between six to nine months and continued stretching, taping, and strengthening are imperative. Infants need to establish correct muscle length tension from midline alignment. This will allow for appropriate firing patterns, range of motion, sequences of movement, adaptive and anticipatory responses and integration of the sensory system.

Adjunctive treatment interventions for torticollis include the following:
- Stretching to SCM, upper trapezius, scalenes, cervical flexors and extensors and trunk
- Scapular mobilization
- Myofascial release
- Soft tissue release
- Cranio-sacral therapy

- Massage: including brushing and light compression
- Strengthening overlengthened muscles
- Splints/bracing: TOT collar, soft cervical collar, helmet for plagiocephaly
- Positioning supports: foam wedge, Boppy noggin nest
- Gravity assisted positions to facilitate stretch and midline

Positioning and handling should focus on midline postural control and symmetry. The visual system may be used to orient the child to postural alignment and to facilitate neck rotation. Supine with head in midline using foam or support wedge, sidelying on the opposite side, pronelying with head turned toward tight SCM, and side carry to lengthen SCM are all positioning options. Strengthening of overlengthened muscles, as well as trunk muscles and scapular stabilizers is key. Focus on symmetrical movement, grading and midline control should be emphasized. Righting and equilibrium responses can be facilitated through weightshifts and transitions.

Treatment duration is determined by the severity of the restriction in range of motion, age at initiation of treatment, and presence of palpable intramuscular fibrotic SCM mass. Conservative management of children with CMT is very successful if initiated prior to two years of age. (Emery, 1994) Goals should include full symmetrical range of motion and mobility, good antigravity neck and trunk strength, symmetrical righting and equilibrium reactions and symmetrical postural alignment.

A thorough medical evaluation is important to rule out other causes for torticollis, prior to the initiation of therapy. X-rays may be indicated. Earlier intervention yields a better outcome and most children will respond well to therapy interventions alone. Helmeting or banding may be required for treatment of accompanying plagiocephaly. Surgery may be required in some cases. The use of Kinesio® Tex tape to assist in the facilitation of specific muscles, as well as to release fascia, muscle tightness and promote optimal alignment is an effective adjunct to the treatment of congenital muscular torticollis and positional torticollis.

Bibliography

American Academy of Pediatrics AAP Task Force on Infant Positioning and SIDS: Positioning and SIDS. Pediatrics 89:1120-1126, 1992

Bratt HD, Merelaus MB; Benign paroxysmal torticollis of infancy; J Bone and Joint Surg Br, May 1992 (vol. 74B) 449-451

Calise E; Treatment Ideas for Pediatric Torticollis; Physical Therapy Forum, May 1991

Canale ST, Griffin DW, Hubbard CN; Congenital muscular torticollis: a long-term follow-up; J Bone and Joint Surgery Am 1982 Jul, 64(7): 810-816

Cheng JC, Tang SP, Chen TM; Sternocleidomastoid pseudotumor and congenital muscular torticollis in infants: a prospective study of 510 cases; J Pediatr. 1999 Jun; 134(6)712-716

Demirbilek S; Congenital muscular torticollis and sternocleidomastoid tumor: results of nonoperative treatment; J Pediatr Surg. 1999 Apr; 34(4)549-551

Dias MS, Klein DM: Occipital plagiocephaly: Deformation or lamboid synostosis? II. A unifying theory regarding pathogenesis. Pediatr Neurosurg 24:69-73, 1996

Golden KA, Beals SP, Littlefield TR, Pomatto JK. Sternocleidomastoid imbalance versus congenital muscular torticollis: Their relationship to positional plagiocephaly. Cleft Palate Craniofacial J., 36 (3); 256-61, May 1999.

Golding-Bird, CH. Congenital wry-neck (caput ostipum congenitale: torticollis congenitalis): with remarks on facial hemiatrophy. Guys Hosp.Rep. 47:253, 1890

Hollier L, Kim J, Grayson BH, McCarthy JG.; Congenital muscular torticollis and the associated craniofacial changes; Plast Reconstr Surg. 2000 Mar;105(3):827-35

Huang et al; The differential diagnosis of abnormal head shapes: separating craniosynostosis from positional deformities and normal variants; Cleft Palate Craniofac J. 1998 May; 35(3):204-211

Huang MH, Gruss JS, Clarren SK, et al: The differential diagnosis of posterior plagiocephaly; True lambdoid synostosis versus positional molding. Plast Reconstr Surg 98:765-774, 1996

Hunt CE, Puczynski MS: Does supine sleeping cause asymmetric heads: Pediatrics 97:877-885, 1996

Kelly KM, Littlefield TR, Pomatto JK, Ripley CE, Beals SP, Joganic EF; Importance of early recognition and treatment of deformational plagiocephaly with orthotic cranioplasty. Cleft Palate Craniofacial J., 36(2):127-130, 1999

Kiesewetter, WB, Nelson, PK, Palladino, VS and Koop, CE. Neonatal torticollis. JAMA 157:1281, 1955

Lidge RT, Bechtol RC, Lambert, CN. Congenital muscular torticollis: etiology and pathology. J. Bone Joint Surg, 39A:1165, 1957

Littlefield TR, Kelly KM, Pomatto JK, Beals SP. Multiple-birth infants at higher risk for development of deformational plagiocephaly. Pediatrics. 103(3): 565-9, 1999

Management of Plagiocephy and Torticollis CSMC Pediatrics/Medical Genetics

Mickelson MR, Cooper RR, Ponseti IV: Ultrastructure of the sternocleidomastoid muscle in muscular torticollis. Clin Orthop 110:11-18. 1975

Mosterman et al; T.O.T. Collar for Effective Management of Torticollis: A New approach to the correction of head tilt in CMT; BCHRF study 1985-1986

Pollack IF, Losken HW, Fasick P: Diagnosis and management of posterior plagiocephaly. Pediatrics 99:180-185, 1997

Powell F; Effects of Kinesio® Taping Method in Treatment of Congenital Torticollis: Case Studies presented at the 15th Annual Kinesio® Taping International Symposium, November, 1999

Rekate HL. Occipital plagiocephaly: a critical review of the literature. J. Neurosurg 89:24-30, 1998.

Seimel-Concepcion J and A. Conway A; "Torticollis Evaluation and Management", presented at Children's National Medical Center Symposium 2000

Task Force on Infant Sleep Position and Sudden Infant Death Syndrome. Changing concepts of sudden Infant Death Syndrome: Implications for infant sleeping environment and sleep position. American Academy of Pediatrics. Pediatrics 105:650-656, 2000

Tien YC, Lin GT, Lin SY; Ultrasonographic study of the coexistence of muscular torticollis and dysplasia of the hip; J Pediatr Orthop. 2001 May-June; 21(3):343-347

Torticollis: Differential Diagnosis, Assessment and Treatment, Surgical Management and Bracing, ISBN 0-7890-0317-1, Karen Karmel-Ross: Published by Haworth Press.

Turk A, McCarthy J, Thorne C, et al: The "Back to Sleep Campaign" and deformational plagiocephaly: Is there a cause for concern?, J Craniofac Surg 7:12-18, 1996

Yu CC, Wong FH, Lo LJ, Chen YR; Craniofacial deformity in patients with uncorrected congenital muscular torticollis: as assessment from three-dimensional computed tomography imaging; Plast Reconstr Surg. 2004 Jan; 113(1):24-33

Resources for therapists and families:

Torticollis: Differential Diagnosis, Assessment and Treatment, Surgical Management and Bracing, ISBN 0-7890-0317-1, Karen Karmel-Ross: Published by Haworth Press.

National Infant Torticollis Association (NITA): http://www.infant-torticollis.org

TorticollisKids.org: http://www.plagiocephaly.org/torticolliskids

Plagiocephaly: http://www.plagiocephaly.org

Boppy pillows: http://www.boppy.com

T.O.T. Collar: http://www.symmetric-designs.com/TOT_collar.html

Plagiocephaly: http://headsupbaby.com

APPENDIX

Patient Name:_____Date:_____

Kinesio® Tex tape is a woven tape that stretches lengthwise. It is made of cotton and does not require the use of an underwrap. Kinesio® Tex tape does NOT contain latex.

Kinesio® Tape can be applied for many reasons. The purpose of this taping technique is:
- ☐ To assist a joint to hold a position, so an overstretched muscle is provided time to shorten. Overstretched muscles are at a disadvantage to work and therefore are often very weak. Once the muscle is given time to return closer to a typical length, it can be recruited for use more efficiently.
- ☐ To provide tactile input and increase proprioception or awareness of a muscle or joint. As sensory awareness increases, more attention is given to an area of the body, which increases use and in turn increases strength.
- ☐ To assist in the release of fascial restrictions or to relax an overused muscle. This allows more optimal alignment and decreased pain in an area.
- ☐ To position a part of the body in better alignment and allow muscles to contract and work in a better position. As these muscles contract in daily activities, they gain strength and control.
- ☐ To decrease swelling, edema and bruising. This will allow for more rapid healing and decreased pain

Wearing Kinesio® Tex tape:
- This tape is a test patch and should be left in place ___ days. It should be removed immediately if any irritation occurs including redness, swelling or itching.
- This tape is a therapeutic treatment and should be left in place ___ days if possible. Please watch the area closely and remove the tape should any irritation occur; including redness, swelling or itching. Remove the tape in time to allow a 24-hour break before returning to therapy to be taped again, or before home reapplication of tape. See attached sheet for application instructions.
- Tape can get wet in pools or baths. Excessive heat will make removal more difficult.
- If tape begins to roll on the edges with wearing, simply trim the edges to prevent them from getting caught on clothes and being pulled off more.

Removal of Kinesio® Tex tape:
- Please take time when removing the tape. Place a thin layer of baby oil, vegetable oil, or tape remover product over the entire area of tape. Let the tape soak for 15 to 20 minutes.
- Loosen one end of the tape and begin slowing peeling the skin away from the tape. Stabilize skin as you move the tape away. Moving in direction of hair growth may cause less discomfort. DO NOT PULL THE TAPE OFF THE SKIN IN A QUICK MOTION. Sometimes removal is easiest in the bathtub.
- After removal, use plenty of lotion to hydrate skin and relieve any irritation. Please do not apply lotion right before re-application of tape, as it decreases the ability of the tape to adhere.

Treating Therapist:_____Phone Number:_____

References

Evaluating the Child for Kinesio® Taping

1. Alexander R, Boehme R, and Cupps B. 1993. Normal Development of Functional Motor Skills: The First Years of Life. Tucson, Arizona: Therapy Skill Builders.
2. Bly L. 1983. The Components of Normal Movement During the First Year of Life and Abnormal Development. Chicago: Neuro-Developmental Treatment Association.
3. Scherzer AL, and Tscharnuter I. 1982. Early Diagnosis and Therapy in Cerebral Palsy –A primer on infant developmental problems. New York, New York: Marcel Dekker, Inc.
4. Kendall FP, McCreary EK, Provance PG, Rodgers MM, and Romani WA. 2005 Muscles –Testing and Function with Posture and Pain 5th Ed. Baltimore,MD: Lippincott Williams & Wilkins.
5. Calais-Germain B. 1993. Anatomy of Movement. Seattle: Eastland Press.
6. Sieg KW, and Adams SP. 1996. Illustrated Essentials of Musculoskeletal Anatomy. Gainesville, Florida: Megabooks, Inc.
7. Cash M. 1999. Pocket Atlas of the Moving Body. London: Ebury Press.

Suggested reading:

Calais-Germain B. 1993. Anatomy of Movement. Seattle, WA: Eastland Press, Inc.

Cusick B. 1997. Legs & Feet: A Review of Musculoskeletal Assessments. (VHS: 2 hrs) Telluride,CO: Progressive GaitWays, LLC.

Kapandji IA. 1982. The Physiology of the Joints 5th Edition- The Upper Limb, Vol 1. New York: Churchill Livingstone.

Kapandji IA. 1988. The Physiology of the Joints 5th Edition-The Lower Limb, Vol. 2. New York: Churchill Livingstone.

Kapandji IA. 1974. The Physiology of the Joints 2th Edition-The Trunk and the Vertebral Column, Vol. 3. New York: Churchill Livingstone.

Kase K, Wallis J, & Kase T. 2003. Clinical Therapeutic Application of the Kinesio® Taping Method. Albuquerque, NM. Kinesio® Taping Association.

Muscolino JE. 2005. The Muscular System Manual-The Skeletal Muscles of the Human Body 2nd Ed. St. Louis, MO: Mosby.

Neumann DA. 2002. Kinesiology of the Musculoskeletal System – Foundations for Physical Rehabilitation. St. Louis, MO: Mosby.

Sahrmann SA. 2002. Diagnosis and Treatment of Movement Impairment Syndromes. St. Louis, MO: Mosby.

Soderberg GL. 1986. Kinesiology Application to Pathological Motion. Baltimore, MD: Williams & Wilkins.

Tachdjian MO.1985 The Child's Foot Philadelphia PA: W.B. Saunders Company

Perry J 1992 Gait Analysis:Normal and Pathological Function New York NY: McGraw-Hill, Inc.

Staheli LT 1998 Fundamentals of Pediatric Orthopedics Philadelphia PA:Lippencott-Raven

Taping Guidelines

Mussehi, J (2003). Experts: Makeup and Skincare. Retrieved from http://experts.about.com/q/1434/3262001.htm

Magnesia Mud Mask. (n.d.). Bottle of rain: a site on home, garden, health, cooking, collecting and everything else. Retrieved from http://bottleofrain.blar.org/bottleofrain.pl?user_record=%2255%22

Phillips Milk of Magnesia. (2004). Retrieve November 12, 2004, from http://kdkaradio.com/content/

content.cgi?database=Logue%20Content.db&command=vi

Brattain, E. (n.d.). Nursery Tips Nappy/Diaper Rash. Retrieved from http://www.hintsandthings.co.uk/nursery/tips.htm

Carpal Tunnel Syndrome
Cailliet R. (1982). Hand Pain and Impairment. Philadelphia: F.A. Davis Company.

Thumb
Napier JP. 1952. The attachments and function of the abductor pollicis brevis. J of Anatomy. 86:335-341.

Weathersby HT, Sutton LR, and Krusen UL. 1963. The kinesiology of muscles of the thumb: An electomyographic study. Archieves of Physical Medicine and Rehabilitation.
June, 321-326.

Palmar Stability
Long, C., et al. (1970) Intrinsic-extrinsic muscle control of the hand in power grip and precision handling. The J of Bone & Joint Surg, 52-A, (5), 853-867.

Radial Digital Grasp
Case-Smith J and Pehoski C. 1992. Development of Hand Skills in the Child. Rockville,MD: The American Occupational Therapy Association, Inc.

Henderson A, and Pehoski C. 1995. Hand Function in the Child- Foundation for Remediation. St. Louis, MO: Mosby-Year Book, Inc.

Elbow
Basmajian, JF and Latif A. (1957). Integrated actions and functions of the chief flexors of the elbow: A detailed electromyographic analysis. J Bone Jt. Surg. 39A: 1106-1118.

Abdominals and Lower Extremity
Cusick B. 1997. Legs & Feet: A Review of Musculoskeletal Assessments. (VHS: 2 hrs) Telluride,CO: Progressive GaitWays, LLC.

APPENDIX

content.cgi?database=Logue%20Content.db&command=vi

Brattain, E. (n.d.). Nursery Tips Nappy/Diaper Rash. Retrieved from http://www.hintsandthings.co.uk/ nursery/tips.htm

Carpal Tunnel Syndrome
Cailliet R. (1982). Hand Pain and Impairment. Philadelphia: F.A. Davis Company.

Thumb
Napier JP. 1952. The attachments and function of the abductor pollicis brevis. J of Anatomy. 86:335-341.

Weathersby HT, Sutton LR, and Krusen UL. 1963. The kinesiology of muscles of the thumb: An electomyographic study. Archieves of Physical Medicine and Rehabilitation. June, 321-326.

Palmar Stability
Long, C., et al. (1970) Intrinsic-extrinsic muscle control of the hand in power grip and precision handling. The J of Bone & Joint Surg. 52-A, (5), 853-867.

Radial Digital Grasp
Case-Smith J and Pehoski C. 1992. Development of Hand Skills in the Child. Rockville,MD: The American Occupational Therapy Association, Inc.

Henderson A, and Pehoski C. 1995. Hand Function in the Child- Foundation for Remediation. St. Louis, MO: Mosby-Year Book, Inc.

Elbow
Basmajian, JF and Latif A. (1957). Integrated actions and functions of the chief flexors of the elbow: A detailed electromyographic analysis. J Bone Jt. Surg. 39A: 1106-1118.

Abdominals and Lower Extremity
Cusick B. 1997. Legs & Feet: A Review of Musculoskeletal Assessments. (VHS: 2 hrs) Telluride,CO: Progressive GaitWays, LLC.